The mature imagination

The mature imagination

Dynamics of identity in
midlife and beyond

Simon Biggs

Open University Press
Buckingham · Philadelphia

Open University Press
Celtic Court
22 Ballmoor
Buckingham
MK18 1XW

email: enquiries@openup.co.uk
world wide web: http://www.openup.co.uk

and
325 Chestnut Street
Philadelphia, PA 19106, USA

First Published 1999

A catalogue record of this book is available from the British Library

ISBN   0 335 20102 4 (pbk)   0 335 20103 2 (hbk)

Library of Congress Cataloging-in-Publication Data
Biggs, Simon, 1955–
    The mature imagination: dynamics of identity in midlife and
    beyond / Simon Biggs.
        p. cm.
    Includes bibliographical references and index.
    ISBN 0–335–20103–2. – ISBN 0–335–20102–4 (pbk.)
    1. Gerontology. 2. Aged – Psychology. I. Title.
HQ1061.B529   1999
    306.26 – dc21   98–33196
                                                                CIP

Typeset by Graphicraft Limited, Hong Kong
Printed in Great Britain by St Edmundsbury Press Ltd,
Bury St Edmunds, Suffolk

To Doreen, Clare, Eve and Guy

Contents

Acknowledgements

The author would like to thank Chris Phillipson and Mike Hepworth for their comments on this manuscript and related material, Michael Allen for ideas and conversation, and Clair Chinnery for her help in preparing graphic material. Thanks also go to Clare Allen and Guy and Eve Biggs for their support and forbearance.

Introduction

WHAT IS THE MATURE IMAGINATION?

To encounter the mature imagination raises issues that are key to both personal and social understanding. How far, for example, is it possible to discover an authentic subjectivity for adulthood? What are the influences that shape our understandings of age and identity? What are the possibilities for change, and how desirable is it perceived to be? In the attempt to answer these and related questions, the reader is invited to take a journey through some of the guiding ideas and assumptions of our times. Contemporary Western societies have developed notions and methods that mould both our conception of the human condition and our perception of the options and alternatives available to us. Chief among them are the psychotherapies and the adoption of lifestyles which are intended to determine the direction of the adult lifecourse. They not only provide, with varying degrees of success, techniques for the modification of body and identity, they also create narratives for the experience of self that allow us to recognize it in certain forms and not others.

But what is meant by mature imagination? The phrase has been adopted in part because there is currently an absence of ways of describing human development in maturity that are positive and offer the prospect of critical analysis. It constitutes a way of approaching the years in which people consider themselves to have reached a level of sustained experience and a certain competence in negotiating adulthood. It includes life-phases that have been described as ranging through midlife and then on into later life and old age. As such, it contains most of the adult lifecourse under contemporary conditions. When one is on its threshold, mature age appears disconcertingly without maps to guide us. The confusion experienced with the approach of maturity has been recognized from the most distant awakenings of the modern period:

> Midway upon the journey of our life,
> I found myself within a dark forest,
> Where the right road was wholly lost and gone.

When Dante wrote this first stanza of the *Divine Comedy*, in 1307, he was 35, the middle-point of the biblical lifecourse, which, it was assumed, spanned three score years and ten. He was, in other words, in midlife, and may have been suffering something of a crisis. The signposts that had allowed him to negotiate the first half of his life had become lost and obscure. There was, on the basis of previous experience, no way out of the wood, except of course, downward. It seemed from the perspective of midlife that one now had to abandon all hope.

Questions about the development of a mature identity – that is to say, an identity that will be serviceable and take the bearer through to deep old age – are of particular contemporary importance. This is not simply because Western societies are in the grip of continued demographic change, but also because a consideration of mature ageing now has a special practical and theoretical value. New ideas are needed to shape the way in which policy-makers, professional helpers and the person in the street think about their own mature years and those of others. A deeper understanding of adult ageing, so long eclipsed by a cultural preoccupation with novelty, childhood and youth culture, can inform our understanding of the contemporary world. Our everyday as well as our formal theories of life, which we often take as givens and rarely subject to critical review, are challenged by ageing. Ageing forces the perception of different paths out of the forest.

A paradox emerges when the words mature and imagination are brought together, which goes to the heart of the issue of identity in adulthood proper. Maturity is couched in the language of completion. One is, at this part of the life phase and according to the *Oxford English Dictionary* (1973), 'fully developed in body and mind', 'complete, perfect or ready'. Dictionaries are good guides to the assumptions of dominant cultures. Here we discover age dressed in the language of completion and fullness. However, flipping backwards to imagination raises a series of different issues. Imagination invites the 'forming of mental concepts of what is not present to the senses . . . beyond those derived from external objects'. It is a imbued with a sense of becoming, of travelling beyond the immediate and the concrete. One imagines other worlds. However, here lies a cultural problem: the questions of mature adulthood are from that part of the lifecourse that many would wish to ignore, to put back on the shelf. They ask about attempts that can be made to make sense of this contradiction between the apprehension of completion and the promise of further and deeper personal development. The issues that ageing raises for culture and an understanding of culture are, more often than not, couched in negative terms as a thing to be avoided, denied or rejected. Identity is a close relation to these concerns. It describes the way in which people present an acceptable face to their social worlds, something that is constructed and maintained, is an act of self-invention which also depends upon social context. It is, then, very much a concept at the crossroads of the personal and the social. It includes within itself props and associations that already exist in the social world, plus ideas, fantasies and desires that arise from an individual's inner being. Some theorists have approached the problem of identity in maturity through the perspective of decline, others through an appreciation of lifestyles that maintain values and assumptions from other parts of the lifecourse; others still have asked about the existential dilemmas that require resolution for a more complete notion of self to emerge. In our journey out of the wood, we are not, then, starting from scratch. Some paths have already been traced through the undergrowth, which, with various degrees of success, suggest where the lifecourse may be heading and in some cases challenge the proposition of thinking in terms of lifecourse at all.

In order to clarify some of these pathways, the chapters in this book have been organized into a series of couplets. First, mature imagination is approached through an examination of the influence of psychoanalysis. As this tradition has developed, increasingly specific and often opposing conceptions of the lifecourse have taken shape. Most notable among these have been the growth of ego psychology in the United States and analytic psychology in Europe, whose influence is felt in a wide diaspora of therapies, models and approaches to ageing. Both are marked by alternative responses to an emerging tension between social conformity and self-expression. Second, consideration is given to postmodern conceptions of contemporary adulthood. Ageing presents a significant challenge to postmodern perspectives on identity, insofar as it suggests a barrier to the possibilities of continual cultural consumption and personal reinvention. The mature imagination, it is suggested, is required to engage in the performance of masquerade, in order to negotiate a series of uncertain options for contemporary identity. While postmodern theorizing appears to eschew metaphors of depth and surface in human experience, these have to be reconsidered in order to make sense of the contradictory circumstances of the ageing identity. Third, special attention is given to the idea of midlifestyle as a solution to some of the problems raised by these different philosophical traditions. Midlifestyles consist of the maintenance of the priorities of mid-adulthood and have been closely associated with ideas that identities can be consumed and invented, depending on immediate circumstances. It is suggested that these lifestyle solutions to the problem of ageing effectively address the surfaces of mature identity but do not question what occurs beyond this social mask. Deeper layers of development therefore need to be engaged with. Fourth, and finally, two chapters are used to explore the relationship between social and personal meaning through the metaphor of social space. Certain spaces may allow the inner and outer logics of mature identity to flow together, while others inhibit this process. The impact of contemporary trends in social policy is considered in case examples of the interaction between socially engineered spaces and the possibilities and desires that the mature imagination might come to contain.

THE ARGUMENT

From psychoanalysis to the active imagination

Our journey to discover an authentic subjectivity for mature adulthood begins with a consideration of the legacy left by the classical psychoanalysis of Sigmund Freud (1905). Psychoanalysis has not only influenced the possibility of therapeutic intervention in maturity, but become something of a cultural icon, infiltrating our everyday common-sense understandings of the human condition. It contains many of the characteristics that have since been associated with modernism, which in this context include an attempt to master the past and a belief in personal progress. Two trends have particularly influenced its perspective on the mature imagination. First and foremost is a focus on childhood as a factor determining the shape of adult identity. Second is a preoccupation with the relationship between hidden parts of the self and the surface meanings attributed to events. From an inauspicious start, in which it was suggested that the sheer volume of material accumulated across the lifecourse and an absence of motivation precluded therapy with mature adults, a succession of revisions threw new light on the ageing psyche. Most importantly, chronological age was unpeeled from an internal experience of how old one felt.

Responses to the Freudian legacy can be seen in the work of Erik Erikson and Carl Gustav Jung, both of whom attempted to understand development across the lifecourse as a whole. Erikson (1959) explored the relationship between social expectation and the key tasks for mature identity, and in so doing asserted the centrality of whichever stage an individual was currently in. However, it is argued that in his attempt to link adult identity to generativity, we are little closer to understanding the unique features of a mature imagination. Indeed, it becomes a series of 'Chinese boxes' whereby whatever stage one looks in for authentic self-expression, the answer lies elsewhere. Jung (1931), on the other hand, saw social conformity and a focus on childhood experience as factors inhibiting personal development. His split with Freud resulted in an entirely different series of priorities being suggested for what he called 'the second half of life'. Central to these ideas was the development of an 'active imagination', which was seen as part and parcel of the adult task of individuation. Mature adults, it is argued, respond to feelings of getting stuck in midlife by discovering previously suppressed potential and engaging in an active dialogue with material from the unconscious. Mature adulthood is thus seen as a time for a natural expansion of the self, in contrast to the constraining presence of social expectation. The enduring view that emerges is of an expanded mature self existing within a hostile social environment.

Choosing not to grow old

Notions of ageing have been radically affected by postmodern conceptions of identity. A heady combination of consumer culture and a need to be constantly recycling a sense of who one is suggests that it may be possible to choose not to grow old. Indeed, personal continuity and a sense of embeddedness in the lifecourse may have become outmoded concepts in what appears to be a continuous enticement from the possibilities presented by contemporary Western societies. Consumer lifestyles have even challenged the restricting presence of the ageing body, now offered reinvigoration at a price, through the use of pharmacology such as Viagra and hormone replacement therapies, a cyborgic merging of bodies and machines and the prospect of genetic engineering. Psychodynamic thinking has itself responded to these changing circumstances by encouraging the peeling of different meanings away from one another. Dependency and old age, chronological age and the personal experience of ageing, social expectation and lifecourse development have all been loosened up in such a way that meanings previously assumed to be coterminous and inseparable may now be distinguished one from another. These trends have been noticeable in a renewed emphasis on the importance of relationships, a focus on the here-and-now and the possibility of multiple identities being contained within the personal psyche. However, it is argued that these trends have privileged surface meanings of identity at the expense of a sense of depth to the personality and the value of history.

Enthusiasts of postmodernity suggest that the increasing uncertainties and rapid changes that are endemic to contemporary social existence should be seen as an opportunity rather than a threat. Baudrillard (1990) has, for example, suggested a world of floating signifiers in which identities can be put together and consumed without reference to the original meanings that different props and attributes might have had. These and other ideas have been employed by writers such as Featherstone and Hepworth (1989, 1995) to examine the possibilities for postmodern ageing. Ageing is considered as a series of progressive betrayals that let an individual down and come between the self and the multiple identities made available through consumerism. We are really, according to this view, all youthful inside, but have become trapped in ageing bodies. The blurring of identity, plus the possibility of prosthetic enhancement and pharmaceutic manipulation of the body, hold out, however, the promise of an indefinite postponement and possible escape from the consequences of ageing.

Ageing also suggests a point at which the postmodern desire to live in a continuous present and see the world as a series of infinitely malleable surfaces hits the buffers of fixity and finitude. There are, in other words, important questions about the human condition that cannot be bucked and which an apprehension of maturity brings into sharper focus.

Maturity and masque

Two starkly different views of the mature imagination are beginning to emerge. First, there is a need to protect development from midlife onwards from a series of negative associations and uncertainties if an inner sense of personal value and integrity is to be preserved. However, there is, second, an awareness of the possibility of creating surfaces for identity, through consumerism and a reversibility of choices that might free mature experience from the coercive hold of traditional stereotypes. It is suggested in Chapter 4 that, in order to understand the development of identity in maturity, both of these processes need to be taken into account. In other words, maturity approximates a masquerade in which certain parts of the self are expressed through the adoption of a persona, a socially acceptable mask, while others are hidden beneath it. This layering of the mature imagination allows identity to be displayed through a cohesive, and thus believable, surface performance which, so to speak, 'gets you through the day'. It exists in episodes and can be modified as circumstances dictate. Indeed, it might be thought of as a signature of maturity that surface identities become malleable and can be used as needed, rather than being too firmly fixed in place or determined by social conformity. The surface performance therefore largely conforms to an external logic, in the sense that it forms a bridge between inner desire and social connection. Beneath this surface of persona and masquerade lies an inner logic that is thereby protected from external attack. The internal logic of maturity would contain a sense of continuity of the self and a relatedness to history that has otherwise been eclipsed. It is here that possibilities and potential that cannot find a place in such an indeterminate world exist and flourish. The mature imagination is therefore conceived of as multilayered. It has the potential of breadth in its surfaces, yet depth in the different layers of psychological expression that it contains.

Midlifestyles

Midlife has become a crossroads for many of these conflicting ideas about the lifecourse. Historically it has been seen successively as a crisis, as a transition and as a lifestyle in and of itself. It is a period of life which is rich in paradox as the increasing certainties of the body's fallibility are apprehended and it is realized that there is no infinite amount of time available to pursue all of one's desires in life. However, it is also a time of increased uncertainty as one becomes simultaneously aware of the precarious nature of existence. Midlife therefore becomes a search for solutions to the puzzling notion of finitude. In the middle of the twentieth century middle adulthood came to be associated with metaphors of crisis (Neugarten 1968). Paradoxically, in order to continue to conform to society's demands, the middle aged were expected to relinquish the goals and identities that had served them well in achieving an acceptable social position. Rebellion was an expected phase that mature adults went through on the road to disengagement and a handing over to the next generation. It was, as has been argued by contemporary social theorists, functional for society; but not functional for the individual at that age.

In the search for an explanation of midlife discontinuity, other periods of transition in the lifecourse were also examined and analogies drawn that helped to explain the midlife experience. Midlife was seen as a recapitulation of adolescent crises of identity (King 1980). But now the mask had become too fixed, and needed to rediscover its flexibility. A heady mixture of changing social expectations, psychological priorities and narcissism.

Midlifestyle can be seen as the latest in this line of metaphors, through a recourse to the salving balm of postmodern reinvention of the self. There are now a multiplicity of cultural images of age that can be employed in the manufacture and consumption of mature identities. Narrative therapies (McAdams 1993) are well suited to this role and have been used specifically to create new lamps out of the old identities that individuals have collected to date. They are the technologies of self invention in mid-life.

A challenging and seductive solution to the ambivalences of midlife can be found in the growth of midlife manuals. These popular writings contain recipes for the maintenance of midlifestyles into an indefinite personal future, a means of positively construing the different phases that mature adulthood supplies and even ways of escaping the ageing process altogether. Rather than harking back to the storms and anxieties of adolescence, this search for a golden age of the youthful self lies in the carefree days of pre-adolescent latency. Narratives are supplied by which one can live through maturity without becoming old. However, it is argued that such narratives have become disconnected from wider issues of authenticity in terms of the lifecourse and of sociability. They are therefore very much a surface phenomenon which leaves many of the difficult questions, that arise through the emergence of a mature imagination, unaddressed.

The mature imagination, it is argued, has to take two processes of identity formation into account. First, a convincing narrative has to be constructed in the here and now, and it is here that it connects with the discourse on surfaces and postmodernity. However, it also has to connect with those increasingly pressing questions that arise with continued ageing, which may not be able to be overtly expressed. Something must exist behind and beyond the masquerade of midlifestyle. If midlifestyle is left to its own devices it increasingly inhabits a world of its own creation, with its own logic that abjures connection with deeper issues of lifecourse development. If the presentation of self is not grounded in these other issues it can almost become psychotic in its reliance on a cut off yet internally consistent world view. Candidates for what is hidden behind midlifestyle appearances are varied and, depending upon circumstances, might include the following. First, a sense of personal continuity through the valuing of memory and the recognition that the remembered past has a life and value of its own, independent of attempts to reconstruct it in the service of current narratives. Second, an apprehension of existential questions arising from the finite nature of life and an associated interest in spirituality. These questions invite the consideration of meanings that transcend the individual, of connection to something greater than the self. This desire for connection also extends to a third area that includes forms of sociability, sexuality, generativity and social action.

The mature imagination is increasingly seen to consist of a complex interplay between depth and surface, from which a variety of possibilities for self-expression and personal identity can emerge. It is suggested that a coming together of depth and surface, of continuity and cohesion, also draws attention to the relationship between reflection and reflexivity. Reflection suggests a reconnection with longitudinal components of identity, the past and future possibility. It rescues an opportunity to stand back and see patterns in events over time. Reflexivity allows a critical apprehension of the present. Imprecision has led to a conflation of these two important processes. Both are needed to achieve a mature awareness of self.

Utopias and dystopias

The argument so far would suggest a changing balance between hidden and surface elements of a mature imagination. For what, in other words, can a voice be found and under what circumstances?

The possibility of genuine self-expression arises when external circumstances and the internal logic of the psyche overlap sufficiently to let
deeper layers of personal concern show through. In order to explore this
relationship further, the qualities of social space have been explored in
more detail. When certain social spaces emerge that are facilitative to
self-expression, reliance on masquerade may be reduced. However, when
the expression of personal identity jars with external, and in this case
age-structured, social meanings, it becomes increasingly layered into tacit
and explicit components. If the social space is hostile to the development
of age-related personal expression, it is possible that what the external,
observing other sees bears little resemblance to internal logic and desire.
The degree to which masking will reduce and internal logic and desire will
become explicit therefore has considerable implications for communication
with helping professionals, the assessment of service quality and forms
of participation.

Following insights from the study of psychodynamic systems in organizational culture, it appears that a key component of facilitative social
space is an ability to contain reflection. By this is meant the degree to
which particular groups, agencies and policies allow protected spaces to
emerge. These protective and facilitative spaces act as a psychological
container for thoughts and feelings that would otherwise not find a voice
in that environment. A social space does not necessarily have to correspond with a particular physical setting or organizational structure, however, and can be extended to include the sorts of meanings that exist
around concepts such as midlife, ageing, old age, health and welfare. The
point is that the shape a space takes is a dynamic pattern of influences
that can either restrict or enhance mature imagination.

Health and social care systems have been key influences on how ageing is shaped within contemporary Western societies. Midlifestyles have
come to dominate identities for those with the psychological, social and
economic resources to engage significantly with age-related consumer
cultures. Recourse to health and social care remains a determining factor
in shaping notions of vulnerability and control that not only affect those
people in need, but spread out to influence the understanding and positioning of later life in wider society and in the public mind. However,
this anchoring point for an ageing identity has been eroded by turn of
the millennium social policy in Europe, Australasia and North America.
In these countries, concern has been raised about the emergence of 'no care
zones' (Estes *et al.* 1993), such that older adults cease to have services
provided to them, where the safety net has been withdrawn altogether.
In some cases it may be that adult ageing provokes entry into 'no identity
zones' (Phillipson and Biggs 1998). These would be social spaces that no
longer contain possibilities for the expression of not simply the active
imagination and existential questions related to adult ageing, but the

possibility of any voice for the requirements of age. Within a century, social policy has moved from a position in which ageing has been over-determined by notions of dependency and disengagement, to a situation in which few if any containing spaces protect mature identity from the vertiginal uncertainties and foreclosing imperatives of contemporary life.

Policy spaces

This is not to say that certain social spaces have failed to emerge as a result of successive policy fashions. Each in its turn, the postwar consensus on state welfare, marketization and, latterly, a social democratic focus on social inclusion and communitarianism, can be interpreted as an attempt to increase the possibilities for personal and social expression. Each includes a different balance between positive containment, as expressed in the possibility for protected, reflective identity and the construction of negative, restrictive spaces in which mature identity must be suppressed. Each has constituted an attempt to shape the nature of citizenship and the place of mature identity within it. It is suggested that two social spaces are opening up in the public mind as we enter a new millennium, both of which are concerned with creating a paradoxical sense of togetherness between workers and those who use human services. The spaces created are often, however, highly ambivalent.

The first of these capitalizes on that sense of uncertainty and flexibility surrounding established social roles, both informal and professional. Trends towards partnership between professional groupings and between those who receive, provide and purchase services blur traditional role boundaries and allow the possibility of recombination. Interprofessional collaboration and user participation, as these trends have been labelled, emphasize the achievement of partnership as a means of combatting social exclusion. It is unclear, however, how far they can include forms of vulnerability which do not fit the partnership model.

The second space presents a disconcerting preoccupation with control and surveillance as a solution to questions of mental capacity, vulnerability and abuse. The abuse of vulnerable adults appears to be a phenomenon that has only recently been formally recognized, and has been recognized under specific policy conditions. While creating a space in which abuse can be discussed and ending an era of silence, swallowed hurt and injustice, it has also, together with a debate on mental incapacity, emerged as a space in which those who do not fit into conceptions of capacity and partnership can be contained.

A continuing theme in both developments is the shaping of mature identity as becoming 'one-of-us', which in this context includes new interpretations of becoming like, of adopting professional mentalities, while at the same time evacuating threats to or dissent from what at first inspection appear as emancipatory spaces.

This discussion of the possibilities for mature imagination raises a number of issues for the social psychology of ageing and the uses of psychotherapy, lifestyle and medical technology. It suggests new directions for research and service development. Most importantly, it breathes life into the human condition in midlife and beyond.

1

Maturity and its discontents

THE POWER OF PSYCHOANALYSIS

It would be foolish to begin a book on mature identity without consider-
ing the powerful role played by psychoanalysis. Psychoanalytic thinking
has not only held a key position in shaping how identity is conceived,
but also helped to form contemporary notions of what it is to be an adult
and the role of ageing in the scheme of things. It has influenced and in its
turn been influenced by views of the self and identity from the beginning
of the twentieth century through to the present, and exemplifies many of
the changes that have come about in how we think, feel and act concerning the mature imagination.

As a leading theoretical position of the modern world, psychoanalytic
ideas have entered everyday life and become part of the way we think
and interpret our experience of the social world. This influence has been
particularly strong among the helping professions in health and social
care. Here, the medium in which work takes place concerns people and
their problems, and the means of achieving change depends to a large
extent on attitudes, values and personal skills. A theoretical position that
prioritizes the hidden influences on motivations of workers no less than
patients, clients and other users of services, plus the relationship between
mind, body and society, is of considerable import to the core concerns of
this area. The cultural embeddedness of psychodynamic thinking means
that it often forms a tacit conceptual backdrop, lending shape to rules of
thumb used by practitioners to make sense of issues in their day-to-day
work. The impact of the psychodynamic tradition can be felt in at least
three ways: as a therapeutic tool, as a source of personal narrative and as
a cultural phenomenon in its own right.

First, then, psychoanalysis and other psychodynamic approaches can be
understood as a therapeutic endeavour aimed at achieving specific curative

results. Here, the psychodynamic approach refers to a particular method of achieving change in troubled individuals, of which psychoanalysis, the method developed by Sigmund Freud and his followers, was the first and most influential. These methods have been referred to as the 'talking therapies', as it is through discussion rather than through medical or drug therapy that change is achieved. They have also been called 'depth therapies', as they rely on the uncovering of meanings which are considered to underlie everyday thought, emotion and action. As such, they could be thought of, to use a Foucauldian (1977) term, as 'technologies of the self', a means by which personal identity can be altered in one direction or another through the application of certain techniques applied by suitably trained initiates. However, once a method has become established, there is a tendency for practitioners to apply that technology, uncritically, to different persons or groups of people (Rustin 1991), with perhaps too much concern as to whether these persons and groups fit the method, rather than it being adapted to new conditions. Work with mature adults, for example, could then be seen as an extension of the method to another area, often marginal to the main concerns of the discipline, a sort of conceptual imperialism whereby increasingly exotic and macabre aspects of the human condition come within its sway. It is questionable whether sufficient attention is given, under such conditions, to the diverse responses and specific needs of mature and older adults. This is not to deny that practitioners genuinely wish to help older adults and are courageous in their attempts to do so. Such an interest has given rise to questions about the effectiveness of certain approaches with older people and the special phenomena that this work uncovers (see, for example, Knight 1986; O'Leary 1996; Terry 1997). These and similar considerations will be addressed by the current investigation, insofar as they bear on the subjectivity of mature adulthood and the shaping of midlife and old age that results.

Second, a psychodynamic understanding of the world supplies a narrative that can be used for the construction of a personal story or identity. Even if one is not engaged in psychotherapy as a method, the tradition and the whole way of thinking that comes with it can influence the way the lifecourse is interpreted. Psychoanalysis provides a framework within which personal events can be made sense of as part of a broader story. The tradition of explaining daily life in terms of psychoanalyic theory is a long one, as exemplified by Freud's (1901) work *The Psychopathology of Everyday Life*, which attempted to display the hidden meanings of common behaviours, and in the process introduced an unsuspecting world to the 'Freudian slip'. Succeeding descriptions of human development, such as Erikson's (1959) eight psycho-social stages of the life cycle, prioritize certain experiences and interpret events within a particular framework. Some aspects of the lifecourse are thereby seen as more important than others, and are differently situated in terms of conceptual importance. If, for example, a young person experiences anxiety over how to dress for a friend's party, to present oneself to a social audience, an Eriksonian framework might locate that experience as part of a preparation of an adult social role, while a more traditional psychoanalytic interpretation would focus on a displaced expression of unresolved sexual attraction within the family. How an event is evaluated and what is done about it depends on how it is seen as fitting into such a wider narrative. These theories provide potential frameworks for the whole lifecourse and the shape and value attributed to different phases. Midlife, for example, may be presented as a new beginning or as an adjustment to decline. Each will influence the stories people tell themselves about their own and others' life experience.

Third, psychoanalysis exists as a cultural phenomenon independently of its use as a method of change or personal understanding. When Freud (1930) wrote *Civilization and Its Discontents* he imagined that he was applying the psychoanalytic method in order to explain social phenomena, as a showcase for the theoretical power of psychoanalysis. Civilization, as he referred to Western societies of the time, became an object of study, another case example. However, psychoanalysis also influences the culture that it is a part of as a cultural phenomenon in its own right. Over time it transforms its own objects of study and is, at the same time, transformed by them. People begin to use and identify with ideas originating from psychoanalysis because they have simply become part of the language of individualistic Westernized cultures. The assumptions held within psychodynamic thinking become part of the common-sense world maintained by those cultures. This taken-for-granted ragbag of tacit assumptions binds a cultural world view together. In other words, we don't have to think about them any more as they become part of the assumed foundations on which everyday decisions can be based. With the domestication of these once radical ideas, observations that were shocking and transformative become commonplace and lose the power to disturb. It is not even necessary to know where these assumptions originated any more, they are just there. Such assumptive realities are fine when we use them as fleeting explanations for why we might keep mislaying the keys to our parent's house, but become more problematic when they provide the tacit framework guiding our cultural attitudes towards intergenerational relationships and their value. At this point tacit cultural assumptions influence both the subjectivity of later life and the positioning of those phases of the lifecourse.

PSYCHODYNAMIC APPROACHES AS PART OF MODERNISM

Psychodynamic approaches to the human subject can also be seen as part of a wider trend in Western social thought. They share properties that place them within the 'modern' tradition, arising from the Enlightenment, which includes a belief in progress, the power of rationality and the positive value of individual autonomy. A focus on change and critical stance towards that which has gone before is typical of modernist theories (Frosh 1991). For modernism, the present is temporary, a way station between the restrictions of the past and a utopian future, and a means of snapping the chains linking the present to the past.

In terms of progress, psychoanalysis conceives of human development as an unshackling of the personality from the constraints of a personal history. This process involves the strengthening of the rational ego by extending its power over the chaotic contents of the unconscious. This is said to occur through an archaeology of the mind whereby hidden memories are rediscovered and made available to consciousness. The psychoanalytic method provides a scientific analysis of problems that can lead not only to the uncovering of reality behind appearance, but to an improved lot for individuals now freed in the present. It is, in this sense, a critical eye that banishes past superstitions, shows us the way that the world works and how we can overcome constraint. This approach to personal development shares many characteristics with the social and historical rise of the bourgeois class in eighteenth- and nineteenth-century Europe and the United States – an overthrow of traditional religious and aristocratic power through a privileging of the virtues of work, science and active individualism (Kumar 1995). At bottom, people are responsible for their own well-being and, in lifecourse terms, prudence in a productive adulthood lays the foundations for a satisfying old age. However, psychoanalysis also has an ambivalent relationship to bourgeois social aspiration. The great paradox of psychoanalysis was that in order to increase the circumference of rationality, the domain of the conscious ego, it highlighted the simultaneous presence of the irrational unconscious and the power of sexuality. It was, as Zaretsky (1997) has pointed out, a radical force in the early years of the twentieth century which subverted many of the assumptions held about everyday reality.

Psychoanalysis is particularly important as a personal narrative and cultural signifier of ageing because it is first and foremost a developmental theory. It includes certain assertions about the lifecourse, the possibilities it holds, its scope and direction. It identifies areas that are formative and how those formations then influence subsequent relationships and possibilities. It maintains a view on the past, the present and the future, with the past as key to a psychoanalytic understanding of the lifecourse. Much of the behaviour and identity occurring in adulthood, it is assumed, can be explained through an examination of childhood experience. Further, because of the therapeutic orientation of the approach, the past is also generally seen as being problematic. Relationships that take place in the individual's past, particularly between generations, are given priority of place when explaining difficulties in the present. Thus, while the past is afforded considerable importance, it is also construed negatively. The story that psychoanalysis tells us about human development describes certain persons, or objects of attention, as heroes and others as villains. Significant adults from one's childhood are likely to be positioned as determining the difficulties one has in weathering the contemporary challenges of adult life. As these significant adults, or others who signify them by dint of a shared cohort experience or chronological age, also coexist in the here-and-now, this view implies an attitude towards older adults in general. Whether these older adults are conceived of as receiving the projected associations of parental figures, or come to signify the past itself, there is an associated danger that they become negatively positioned within the world view that the theory represents. Further, because childhood is seen as being formative, it is paid much more attention in theoretical terms than other parts of the lifecourse. Psychodynamic thinking tends, then, to be highly developed in its understanding of the early lifecourse and underdeveloped in its consideration of later phases.

A second core distinction that emerges from the approach concerns the relationship between hidden and surface meanings attributed to personal and social phenomena. Modernism, with its critical interest in 'deep structures' that determine or situate existing surfaces of culture, conceives immediately observed events as a reflection of an underlying reality. To understand and achieve control over the lifecourse, it is necessary to make these tacit substrates explicit. For psychoanalysis, it means that what you see is not what you get. A multiplicity of inner meanings can adhere to any one event and, while these might not be immediately available to consciousness, a method is supplied to uncover them. The distinction between hidden and surface meanings also allows chronological age to be peeled off from psychological age. Thus, while one might be classified for external purposes as 24, 48 or 83, the internal experience of self could be at any of these ages at any one point in time. The experience of disjuncture between internal and external attributions of age has been noted by a number of writers (de Beauvoir 1970; Featherstone and Hepworth 1989; Thompson 1992) and is a key contribution to the study of mature identity. Psychoanalysis supplies a conceptual apparatus for examining the meanings that such an experience might hold. Adopting distinction between the hidden and the surface also allows the possibility that an overt presentation of identity might serve to protect other aspects of the self which are not immediately observable. The process of hiding may be unconscious or contain degrees of conscious awareness. This perspective lends a multilayered quality to human relationships that helps to destabilize stereotypic assumptions about fixed definitions of age and ageing.

The value attributed to past and childhood events, when added to the relationship between hidden and surface meaning, has lead to a particular view of the mature imagination, which we will begin to explore below.

AGEING: AN INAUSPICIOUS START

Freud's initial statements on the prospects for development in mature adulthood are few, and are dispersed among papers that are largely concerned with other issues. Regardless of their peripheral status in Freud's own thinking, these comments have had considerable influence on the subsequent theory and practice of psychoanalysis. Much has been made of an address delivered to the Viennese medical profession in 1904, and published in 1905 as part of his essay *On Psychotherapy*. It is here that he claims: 'psychotherapy is not possible near or above the age of 50, the elasticity of the mental processes, on which treatment depends, is as a rule lacking – old people are not educable – and, on the other hand, the mass of material to be dealt with would prolong the duration of treatment indefinitely.' Freud (1905: C.W. 1953, 7: 264).

Curiously, Freud was himself 48 when he gave his address and thus fell within his own 'near or above' age-range, a period, as Hildebrand (1982) notes, before he entirely recast his own theory of mind, establishing the concept of oedipal conflict and thus the intellectual foundations of psychoanalysis itself. Similarly, many key thinkers in the growth of psychoanalytic thought also began their analyses in their mid to late forties. Melanie Klein was 41 when she began a personal analysis with Karl Abraham, and Wilfred Bion was 48 when he started with Klein (Hinshelwood personal communication, 1998).

It has been suggested that the context in which Freud gave his address might be crucial to his down-playing the value of psychoanalysis in later life. His audience was, according to Knight (1996), regarded as potentially hostile, and as other commentators have noted (Billig 1997), this was a period in which Freud was particularly concerned with social acceptance. Freud was beginning a period of social and professional rehabilitation after the publication of *Studies on Hysteria* with Breuer in 1895, which had provoked a decade of intellectual isolation. In that book, he outlined a possible psychosexual basis to phenomena hitherto thought of as purely physical in origin, and introduced the possibility of a 'talking' therapy. It was thus crucial that the 1904 address was purged of any further unorthodoxy from a speaker whose reputation was closely associated with the propagation of salacious views. The tenor of the paper is cautious, outlining circumstances for the use of psychoanalytic method that 'can scarcely be laid down as yet', and, as part of that caution, Freud suggests conditions under which his new therapy might be inappropriate.

He is playing safe, and rules out 'psychoses, states of confusion and deeply rooted depression' and cases in which the 'speedy removal of dangerous symptoms' is required. Along with that list comes middle and later life.

Mature ageing is cited in only two other notable instances from the entirety of Freud's work. One predates the 1904 speech: *Sexual Aetiology of Neuroses* (1897) is largely speculative, with little evidence that Freud had practical experience with older patients to draw on. It is suggested that psychoanalytic therapy might be unsuitable for the young and the 'feeble minded', as well as people who are 'very advanced in years'. Two main reasons are cited for not using psychoanalysis with this latter group. The first concerns what has come to be known as the argument over accumulated material, and refers to the amount of experience accrued over a lifecourse which, it is argued, would take too long to analyse. The second reason refers to a lack of value attached to 'nervous health' in the later stages of adulthood. Who attaches this lack of value to later life, whether it is the analyst, society or the patients themselves, is unclear from the text.

Further explanation of what might be meant by this assertion can be found in a third reference to later life in Freud's own work, occurring in *Types of Onset of the Neuroses* (1912). In this text, neurotic breakdowns are linked to puberty and the menopause, which themselves are related to 'more or less sudden increases of libido'. It is argued that libidinal energy, which is seen as providing the motor of psychological change with its fuel, is otherwise relatively absent in later life. This absence leads to a pessimistic general prognosis for interventions after the menopause in women, and presumably men at that stage in life. According to this 'classical' Freudian view, 'a combination of the defences of older patients becoming rigid and a reduced drive for libidinal gratification meant that there was unlikely to be sufficient motivation for change in later life' (King 1974: 22). Freud did not, however, make a link between the presence of neurotic conflict that the comments on a menopausal midlife imply, and usually considered the grounds *par excellence* for the employment of psychoanalysis, and the possibility of inducing therapeutic change. He did not, in other words, subscribe to the view, expressed subsequently by Abraham (1919), that it is the age at which a problem appears, rather than the age of the patient, that is of key significance.

It would appear, from the relative absence of source material on later life that occurs in Freud's own writing, that while he might discount the use of psychoanalysis at that point in the lifecourse, these arguments are essentially about technique and only secondly about adult subjectivity. There may be less energy available for psychic change, but there is little to suggest that the mature psyche is not subject to the same processes and mechanisms found in any other part of life. Indeed, an absence of subsequent comment might simply imply the universality of the concepts Freud believed he had discovered.

However provisional and marginal these views appear to be, they quickly gained credence within a growing circle of analysts. This was so much the case that in 1919 Abraham found it necessary to comment that Freud's early opinion 'Is often taken to mean that treatment in the fourth decade of life holds out doubtful prospects of relief, and that in the fifth decade, and particularly in the climacteric, the chances of achieving favourable results are decidedly adverse. Beyond fifty it is often denied that our therapy has any effect at all' (Abraham 1919: 313). Abraham's summary of prevailing opinion seems subject to some chronological slippage itself, as unsuitability now clearly includes midlife. His main point, however, was to defend the use of therapy with older analysands, even though a patient might be 'less inclined to part with a neurosis which he has had most of this life'. For, while longstanding habits might be difficult to change, he summarized four examples of therapeutic work on 'neuroses in persons of over forty and even fifty years of age'. Prognosis, he concluded, depended on age at onset, with earlier onset making the chances of cure less likely. 'In other words the age at which the neurosis breaks out is of greater importance to the success of psychoanalysis than the age at which treatment is begun' (Abraham 1919: 316).

Abraham's commentary seems to have had little impact on an emerging orthodoxy concerning the relationship between psychoanalysis and later life. Rechtschaffen (1959), in what appears to be the earliest review of substance in this area, notes a series of reasons current in the contemporary literature that undercut psychodynamic work in mature adulthood. Among a range of reasoning can be found: reduced ego strength; defences that cannot take the strain; that the older person is thereby too open to self-examination; the undesirability of looking back on the whole of one's life as neurotic and maladjusted; that induced change may not fit with possibilities extant in a patient's external life situation, older people's own reluctance to undertake a kind of treatment which, for cohort reasons, is assumed to be reserved for the mad. He concludes, however, that 'there is no reason to discuss geriatric psychotherapy as distinct from any other psychotherapy, unless there is some assumption that there are, or should be, some distinctive features about it' (Rechtschaffen 1959: 82).

Rechtschaffen's observations on the commonality of work between older and other analysands raise a series of theoretical questions that present an alternative logic of psychoanalysis as it pertains to age. The first of these concerns the view that, regardless of external circumstances, the unconscious is itself timeless. The second concerns the construal of psychological problems as patterns of neurotic repetition. Both of these propositions about the nature of the psyche render arguments based on the accumulated material that older people carry with them unpersuasive. In classical psychoanalysis the unconscious is conceived as essentially without time and chaotic in character. Thus the content and process of unconscious material recovered by the ego is not in itself age-related, although ego processes may subsequently structure it in that way. Further, the key determining period for personal identity occurs in early childhood, with the civilizing resolution of the oedipal crisis. Other conflicts and tensions during the lifecourse are seen as reflections of the attempted resolution of that core determining problem. In other words, in the normal run of things, both the driving force and the patterns and processes for personal psychic equilibrium are more or less set at an early stage and stay that way for the rest of life. Subsequent neurotic experiences are simply repetitions of these early patterns, being played out at other times in the lifecourse. Whatever the material, then, it should evidence patterns that are essentially the same in terms of core psychological processes, however many times those patterns may be re-enacted. The 'mass of material' argument does not hold water, following this logic, because it is the underlying processes that determine the validity of material, and not vice versa. This interpretation would explain the absence of reference to the age of patients in Freud's mature work, as it can reasonably assumed that he saw it as irrelevant.

The argument against work with older people is therefore largely speculative, cautious and clearly not central to psychoanalytic thinking. Curious references to the negative effects of accumulated material may simply be a nod in the direction of ageist attitudes current at the time that Freud was writing. The allusion to reduced libidinal activity is more difficult to dismiss theoretically, since it might obtain empirical support. However, in spite of these remarks in Freud's early writings, which, as we have seen, touch only briefly on the relationship between ageing and psychoanalysis, a legacy has been left that associated the legitimacy of the therapeutic enterprise with caution as to its value in later life. By 1952, Hollender was prompted to note, for example, that 'Perhaps the best explanation for the fact that analysis is not a procedure for people in their fifties and over is that there is not enough hope in the future to provide the motivation needed to endure the tensions mobilised by analysis' (Hollender 1952: 342).

So, arguments concerning the amount of material accumulated over a long life and the absence of mental elasticity may not in themselves be sound. They have, however, contributed to a climate in which it had, by the 1960s, been accepted not only that therapy was ineffective with mature individuals but also that those over 40 should be dissuaded from analytic training. While there is a significant strand of conservatism and 'followership' in this state of affairs, psychoanalysis also shows itself open to an alternative and more subversive perspective. Arguments in Freud's work suggest that as the forces and contradictions that determine personal psychology are unconscious, and formed at an early age, chronological age in adulthood is largely irrelevant to depth psychology. In other words, adult patients should be treated similarly, regardless of age.

REVISING THE DOCTRINE

During the 1960s and 1970s Pearl King's (1974) was one of the few dissenting voices against the dominant view that analysis and maturity were simply not compatible. She argued that 'particularly between the ages of 40 and 65' older patients can benefit greatly from analysis, but because of the prevailing belief system within psychoanalysis, very few older people actually found their way into analysis. King describes a contemporary climate among practising psychoanalysts in which colleagues would only quietly 'confess' to working with patients who were over 40 years old. She failed, however, to get her views accepted within neo-Freudian circles, and had to present her paper to the Jungian Society of Analytical Psychology. This was a time of considerably less eclecticism than the present. Rivalry existed between these two camps, which, as Homans (1995) put it, led to a period in which Freudians and Jungians hated and then just ignored one another.

Regardless of such institutional scepticism, King, her analysand Hildebrand and a small number of other analysts maintained an interest in work with older people. Although this work was often expressed as extending the benefits of psychodynamic treatment to a novel population of patients, it marked a trend beginning to take place across the psychodynamic terrain, which was later to include work with 'borderline personalities' on the boundaries of psychosis (Steiner 1993) and people with learning difficulties (Sinason 1992). Both King (1974) and Hildebrand (1982, 1986) were exercised to show that psychoanalysis can be used with older adults, that psychoanalytic theory can explain a widening lifecourse territory. As such, their approach was both a radical and, in King's time, dangerous departure from neo-Freudian orthodoxy.

Reduced rigidity and transference relations

As part of this process, thinking on the nature of late-life development also began to turn on observations that had previously been used to discount work with older people. The first of these realignments concerned the consequences of lessened libidinal energy, which had proved such a convincing theoretical barrier to work with mature patients. The increased flexibility that had been attributed to a weakening of 'ego-strength' or lessened 'nervous energy' now emerged as an advantage of working psychoanalytically in mature adulthood.

King (1974) drew on the earlier observation (Grotjahn 1955) that whereas the demands of external reality might be perceived by younger adults as a narcissistic threat to their personal identity, older adults were less threatened and would thereby exhibit less resistance to unpleasant insights about themselves. They were therefore more able to integrate therapeutic interpretations. She noted a 'new dynamic and sense of urgency' that mature adults brought to therapy. This sense was not, however, driven by libidinous instinct, but a keener awareness of the finite nature of existence. The lessening of nervous energy 'reduces the need for the maintenance of the rigidity of their defence systems, so that [mature adults] are able to assimilate new objects into their psychic structure ... and they begin to experience a *new sense of their own identity* and the value of their own achievement and worth' (King 1974: 33, italics in original). King uses the language of true and false selves to underscore her argument, so that mature adulthood is seen as constituting a shift from the presentation of a false to a more authentic identity. Hildebrand (1986: 22) also discovered that older patients exhibited 'a good deal of capacity to delay gratification, allow problems to resolve and take the long view. Moreover they often have much greater self-reliance than do younger people and can be left to get on with things by themselves.' According to the revisionists, then, mature adults were less driven by achievement in the external world and more conscious of mortality than younger adults, differences that made them more, rather than less, susceptible to psychodynamic change.

A second realignment concerned the nature of the unconscious associations that the patient and therapist have towards each other, which in psychoanalysis are referred to as transference and counter-transference, respectively. While Rechtschaffen (1959) noted the existence of 'reverse-transference' when a therapist was younger than an analysand, King's (1974) observations on transference phenomena appear to constitute the first serious consideration of adult subjectivities within the psychoanalytic tradition. It is here that psychoanalysis begins to accommodate mature age rather than simply assimilating it into an existing schema.

The importance of transference stems from its status, from the earliest days of psychoanalysis, as the main vehicle through which positive change can occur. This is because it is by re-experiencing early formative events in one's relationship with the analyst, and thereby reworking them, that analysis has its effect. Typically this process would involve an older analyst being seen as the parent of the younger patient, and by working through this relationship afresh and in fantasy form, the patient can learn to outgrow projections based on childhood and adopt a more appropriate adult identity. King (1980: 154) points out, however, that: 'middle aged and elderly clients may be functioning within a number of different timescales. These may include a chronological time scale, a psychological one and a biological one, or unconscious processes which are paradoxically timeless.' The implication of this is that the Other, in terms of transference the analyst, 'can be experienced as any significant figure from the elderly patient's past, sometimes covering a span of five generations, and for any of these transference figures the roles may be reversed' (*ibid.*). Mature patients, in other words, may behave towards the therapist independently of the actual ages involved and in combinations beyond the traditional Freudian view in which analysand equals child and analyst equals parent. Hildebrand (1986) has referred to this process as an 'inverted' transference because older patients are just as likely to respond emotionally to the analyst as a daughter or son as they are as a parent. Knight (1986, 1996), who adopts an eclectic position on psychodynamic theory, indicates that therapists and others may be responded to as if they were the child, grandchild, parent, spouse or lover of an older person, depending upon the quality of their emerging relationship. Further, this may also happen in reverse, so that those working with older people may themselves experience counter-transference such that they act out unconscious associations arising from their own unresolved conflicts with figures from across the lifecourse. These tacit influences, if left unexplored, may explain the resistance of many helping professionals to work with older people (Biggs 1989).

This reformulation of transference phenomena marks a considerable shift in the psychodynamic understanding of intergenerational relations, because it is recognized that both younger and older participants may now inhabit a multiplicity of possible age-related spaces. These identities should, moreover, be valued and not rejected as 'resistances' or as in some way perverse. The extension of transference phenomena across the lifecourse further facilitates the unpeeling of chronological from psychological age and, in so doing, contributes to the deconstruction of common-sense stereotypes of ageing.

The defining presence of childhood

In her paper, King (1980) gives two case examples of patients: a man in his 'early sixties' and a woman in her 'fifties'. Both cases are used to illustrate the idea that life transitions can provoke the reworking of unresolved neurotic conflicts from earlier life phases. 'For middle aged and elderly patients', she states, 'the traumas and psychopathology of puberty and adolescence must be re-experienced and worked through in the transference whatever early infantile material is also dealt with. One reason for this may be that the middle aged individual is having to face many of the same problems as he did in his adolescence, but this time in reverse' (King 1980: 156).

The problems that King refers to include sexual and biological change and changes to social roles and relationships. Each transition contributes to conflicts around dependency and independence. Here, psychological conflict and change is seen as part and parcel of later life. However, a closer reading indicates that change in maturity has been positioned in a particular way. Hidden behind this transitional model is a logic familiar to the neo-Freudian tradition. Mid- and late-life transitions are effectively seen as a third and possibly fourth reworking of early conflicts, the second being maturational and identity transitions in adolescence. Adolescence is itself seen as a 'genital' working through of an original oedipal conflict. The oedipal is thus primary, but resurfaces in different forms at different times over the lifecourse. In this respect King is, at base, presenting a highly orthodox psychoanalytic position, giving little consideration to the unique existential tasks that might face individuals in later life.

References to work with older patients, which are few and far between in the psychoanalytic literature, almost always reflect a focus on conflicts resonant of childhood. Hannah Segal (1958: 174), for example, described the analysis of an elderly man who was thought to be 'unconsciously terrified of old age and death which he perceived as a persecution'. She saw in this anxiety a failure to incorporate ambivalence. This is normally resolved by working through what, in Kleinian terms, would be the psychological transition from a paranoid/schizoid splitting of good from bad to a depressive position in which one can cope with complexity and concern for others. The resolution of both positions is thought to take place in the earliest years of life. Similarly, Nina Colthart (1991), while sensitive to specific features particular to work with older patients, indicates that the core processes underlying psychological distress lead back to childhood experiences. During the analysis of two men, one aged in his seventies, the other in his late fifties to early sixties (analysis taking several years to complete), she considered that early life experiences were relived in 'a remarkable, and condensed way'. Thus, 'The dynamic quality of sequential periods of life resembles a series of plays, with existing characters taking on new roles as the scenarios shift and development takes place' (Colthart 1991: 210).

In summarizing this position it would seem that, whereas the ground on which conflicts take place may change with age, causative factors can be reduced to traditional psychodynamic explanations, based on childhood experience. In explanatory terms, most lifecourse phenomena can be reduced to the primacy of childhood.

THE HIDDEN LEGACY

At this point it is possible to summarize psychoanalytic arguments on the status of ageing (see Figure 1.1). The contention that mature adults

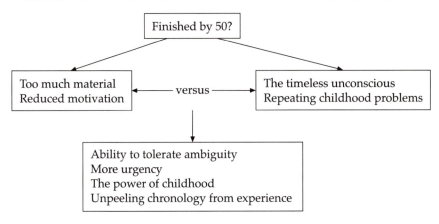

Figure 1.1   Psychoanalysis and the mature imagination.

have too much life experience and are unmotivated can be contrasted with the timelessness of the unconscious and the repetition of personal conflicts. Further development has emphasized a reduced rigidity and greater urgency in later life, while maintaining the central influence of childhood experience.

It appears from this review of the changing relationship between psychoanalysis and adult ageing that the primary contribution to understanding the authentic subjective experience of mid and later life arises from an unpeeling of external referents to ageing, such as chronological age and immediate appearance, from the inner life of the ageing individual. The question of an ageing identity is posed in terms of the hidden and the surface and is most apparent in discussion of intergenerational transference and counter-transference relations. This unpeeling facilitates the awareness of multiple identifications that are based on age and frees the inner life of the active subject from the constraints of social expectation, which in this case can be seen in the traditional psychoanalytic posture of analyst as parent and analysand as child. As a consequence of this observation, it is possible to conceive of age-based identities both as existing independently of the age of the patient and as opening identity management up to the possibilities of explicit and tacit, overt and disguised presentations of self.

The inner world of the mature adult may therefore contain a series of optional age-related identities that come in and out of focus depending upon the circumstances that mature adults find themselves in. The degree of control that can be gained over these possible presentations might depend upon a natural process of psychological maturation or on the practice of psychoanalysis itself, although, perhaps unsurprisingly, supporters of the psychoanalytic method favour the latter interpretation.

The relationship between the overt and the disguised that is being suggested here differs from the original formulation of material hidden in the unconscious versus that made knowable to the ego. Rather, an expansion of this formulation suggests that both the surface and the hidden can be knowable to the subject, such that one knows that one's appearance no longer conveys radiant youth yet one can feel young, old or in between, beyond physical and social constraints associated with age.

However, the continuing disadvantage that emerges from the psychoanalytic literature concerns the reduction of adult problems to their childhood causes. This assertion constitutes a core belief within the psychoanalytic tradition and is unlikely to be changed: indeed, it is likely that there are many adults in midlife and beyond who are still restricted and in some cases mentally tortured by the repetition of the identity issues arising in early childhood. The problem that this poses for an examination of the mature imagination is not insignificant. At a most transparent level, we are told little about the particular subjectivity of mid and late adulthood if this is conceived of as the replaying of oedipal conflicts. The privileging of oedipal identifications means that other processes occurring in the adult psyche are either under-emphasized or simply seen as distractions from the primary objective of reworking that conflict in order to achieve an identity that is more at ease with itself. These other processes are thereby denied voice by the dominant discourse. At a wider, tacit level, the privileging of childhood, even among the most progressive, age-sensitized psychoanalysts, contributes to a construction of late life development as of lesser importance, thus aligning it with other ageist beliefs in contemporary society. Thus, the story that psychoanalysis tells us about mature adulthood is that its centre of gravity lies elsewhere and that change does not depend upon issues and priorities in the present. Indeed, not only is the past privileged as holding the key to current problems, the process of psychoanalysis constitutes a method of liberation from constraints found there.

At the level of shaping mature adulthood, of answering the question of where older adults appear in the plot, they appear as the significant adults of one's childhood. In other words, they come to represent that which must be rejected in the present and are potentially negative contributors to the life phase one is currently in. It is not simply that mainstream psychoanalysis characterizes older adults as difficult in treatment, but that it also positions them as marginal in the world view that it promotes as a potential personal narrative and as a cultural arbiter of social significance. Psychoanalysis leaves an inheritance that is highly ambivalent towards adult ageing. On the one hand, it opens the possibility of multiple internal perspectives on mature identity. On the other, it appears to sideline the subjective experience of ageing, excepting when it can be interpreted in relation to childhood experience.

The story of identity drawn by the psychodynamic tradition does not end with debates within psychoanalysis itself. Two perspectives have drawn on the insights of this approach and have expanded upon adult development in very different ways. It is to them that we now turn.

2

From ego psychology to the active imagination

Two psychodynamic thinkers have influenced contemporary conceptions of mature identity more than any others. Erik Erikson has developed ideas, latent within psychoanalysis, that expand the role of the conscious ego and thereby link the self more closely to the social world. Carl Gustav Jung was principally interested in the development of self-expression in adulthood, and made a clear distinction between the preoccupations of childhood and what he called the 'second half of life'. Both have expanded on the relationship between adult identity and the spaces allotted to it in everyday life.

ERIK ERIKSON AND EGO PSYCHOLOGY

It is hard to over-emphasize the influence of Erikson's theorizing on the lifecourse, which in his later years took the form of a closer examination of later life itself. Sugarman (1986: 83), for example, refers to its 'pride of place when the whole life span is considered'. Erikson's model moved psychodynamic thinking on from a preoccupation with psycho-sexual development to psycho-social adaptation. That is to say, whereas psycho-analysis concerned itself with how the ego might control unconscious drives and impulses, ego psychology, of which Erikson's ideas are a part, paid closer attention to the role of conscious awareness and its relation to social adaptation. This led to a reduced conceptual emphasis on libidinal energy as both a motor for psychological change and a primitive force that needed to be channelled. Instead, Freud's original ideas on the civil-izing influence of the ego were extended, creating an increased role for social expectation as a formative influence on psychological development. This development in psychodynamic theory better fitted the historical and cultural climate that Erikson and other ego psychologists, such as

Fromm (1956) and Horney (1955), found in the post-war society of the United States. In terms of the lifecourse, it led to a growth of interest in consciousness beyond childhood, and thus a more developed view on the position of mature adulthood and old age. It also led to the abandonment of preoccupations with the reduced psychological motivation that European psychoanalysis had come to associate with later life.

The Eriksonian life cycle

The lifecourse, or 'life cycle' as it is called within the model, is seen to consist of eight age-stages, within which a series of psycho-social crises, bipolar conflicts and their resolution determine the form taken by personal development. It is proposed that the stage a person is currently at lends coherence to the perception of preceding and subsequent experience, so that each stage 'is grounded in all the previous ones; while in each the developmental maturation (and psycho-social crisis) of one of these virtues gives new connotations to all the "lower" and already developed stages as well as the higher and still developing ones. This can never be said often enough' (Erikson 1982: 59).

Erikson has, on first examination, replaced the defining power of childhood with something else, that something else being the stage of life that an individual is currently experiencing. The centrality of whichever stage the subject is in adds depth to the different preoccupations that growing individuals exhibit. It helps to explain why elders interviewed in Erikson *et al.*'s (1986) longitudinal study gave little emphasis to or simply ignored events that, at the time of happening, were seen as important and potentially traumatic. This process provides a sense of personal continuity while ensuring the ongoing development of individual identity. The perception of continuity and achievement is important to the Eriksonian scheme of things, and continuity, to be fully functional, must look forward as well as back if it is to lend coherence to the experience of self.

The eight stages contained within the model are infancy, early childhood, the play age, school age, adolescence, young adulthood, adulthood and old age, each with its own special conflict to be negotiated. In adulthood, for example, it is argued that the core tensions that have to be resolved are between generativity and stagnation, and that the conflict that this bipolarity represents concerns an attitude towards caring. In old age, tension is said to exist between integrity on the one hand and disgust and despair on the other. The resolution of this conflict will influence the achievement of wisdom at the end of the lifecourse. It can be seen from these examples that the bipolarities described by Erikson are evaluative in tone, suggesting the nature of a successful outcome at any one stage.

In *The Life Cycle Completed*, Erikson (1982: 55) describes his age-stage model as enumerating the 'Basic qualities that "qualify" a young person to enter the generational cycle – and an adult to conclude it.' This process engages the individual with existing social structures such that a 'Widening radius of interpersonal relations leads, at each stage, to that contact with new sections of the social order, which thus provide, even as they depend on, individual development' (Erikson *et al.* 1986: 39). Kivnick describes the 'eight psycho-social themes as a kind of scaffolding around which people construct their lives, from beginning to end' (Kivnick 1993: 20). There is thus a close association within the model between personal development and the social order, such that the latter gives shape to personal development.

Vaillant (1993) claims empirical support for Erikson's stages across class and gender divides, adding two stages. Career consolidation has been inserted between young adulthood and adult generativity, with a 'keeper of meaning' role appearing between adulthood and old age. The focus here is on the balance that can be achieved as one moves from one stage to another and on 'the developing adult's ego capacity to master and feel at home in an increasingly complex social radius' (Vaillant 1993: 146). 'Career consolidation' therefore 'involves the transformation of pre-occupation with self, of commitment to an adolescent hobby, and of "seeking the bauble of reputation", into a specialised role valued by both self and society' (Vaillant 1993: 146).

Erikson's model has arguably achieved greatest fame from the identification of an adolescent identity crisis. This crisis acts as the formative period for entry into adulthood, and has been elaborated by Marcia (1966). Here, conflict exists between the establishment of a secure or confused identity, involving a process of exploration and commitment, after which one 'achieves identity'. The popularity of Eriksonian views on identity may owe something to the growth of youth culture and associated moral panics that occurred at approximately the same historical period as the publication of his seminal work *Childhood and Society*, first published in 1950 and revised in 1963. Adolescent identity formation is positioned as the gateway into full adulthood. Thus, on closer examination, identity formation is of secondary value within the Eriksonian lifecourse. Its value depends on the degree to which the identity that is fixed creates a stable basis for generativity in work and family life that takes place during the fully adult and generative stage.

At the other end of adulthood, Erikson proposes a conflict variously described as being between wisdom and disdain, and integrity and despair. Both of these bipolar conflicts refer to tensions around a final integration of the personality, which Erikson refers to as 'integrality'. According to this view, the great challenge of late life is to maintain a sense of personal 'integrality', which has been defined as 'a tendency to keep things together' (Erikson 1982: 65). Integrality would seem to include two simultaneous themes: an ability to keep body and soul together in the face of physical ageing and the loss of significant others; and the development of a convincing and coherent life story which sums up an individual's lived experience. In other words, the final life-task consists of the 'acceptance of one's own and only life cycle and of the people who have become significant to it as something that had to be and that, by necessity, permitted no substitutions. It thus means . . . An acceptance of the fact that one's life is one's own responsibility' (Erikson 1963: 98).

Subsequently, interest in integrality has been superceded by the positive but less complex notion of integrity. Rennemark and Hagberg (1997) have attempted to associate particular aspects of personal integrity with the remembrance of different age stages in late life. They have operationalized integrity as 'a sense of coherence in perceived life history', such that a coherent relationship between one's remembered past and present existence is positively related to personal well-being. They found that the stages most cited by elders as being influential were childhood and adolescence. However, elders who were not happy in late life were more likely to relate their current circumstances to the 'adult' stage of generativity. There is, however, a difficulty in posing the defining characteristic of late life as coherence, as an ability to draw the strands of a lifecourse together, because according to the Eriksonian schema this fails to distinguish it from other stages. The process of making sense of one's lived experience from the standpoint of the stage one is in, is, as has been noted above, part and parcel of each stage of development. While this has the advantage of reducing barriers between old age and other parts of the lifecourse, it leaves it with little by way of original qualities. Further, as the eighth and final stage of old age is primarily concerned with making retrospective sense of a lived life and then handing on the lessons learned, it is singularly disadvantaged as a source of coherence. Conceptually speaking, the last phase can only look back. It cannot look forward in terms of personal development.

The problem, as Erikson *et al.* (1986) have seen it, is that 'the fabric of society, the centre, "does not hold" the aged', which is a significant difficulty for a model that relies heavily on psycho-social adjustment to structure the lifecourse. While midlife holds the promise of 'a vivid generational interplay', the final period of Erikson's life cycle concerns the predominantly personal and asocial task of 'existential integrity'. In order to integrate the eighth stage into Erikson's system, some conceptual glue must be found from elsewhere.

Two sources, two means, of psycho-social coherence can be found in the work of Eriksonian thinkers. First, as Erikson *et al.* (1986: 14) point out, preceding stages must be used to structure and prefigure old age. Thus, 'From here on, old age must be planned, which means that mature (and one hopes well informed) middle-aged adults must become and remain aware of the long life stages that lie ahead.' Midlife generativity, with its capability of looking forwards as well as backwards, must lay the foundations for late-life integrity, which, after all, can only look back and engage in what has been characterized as a 'grand wrapping-up' (Biggs 1993a).

Second, Kivnick (1988) has suggested that psycho-social meaning might lie in 'post-maintenance generativity' or 'grand-generativity', which, in her understanding, is closely related to grandparenthood. The purpose of the eighth stage, according to this view, would be to support the core tasks of generativity itself, which lie within the preceding stage. This view has been criticized as both conferring a second-hand meaning to later life and assuming that only a certain form of family relationship can facilitate fulfilment (Biggs 1993). It does, however, solve the problem of establishing a meaningful subjectivity in later life by extending the reach of the activities of the preceding stage.

A number of ego psychologists have devised pathways that help create a meaningful, if second-hand existence in later life. Kivnick (1993: 20) goes on to suggest a programme of improving activities for late-life development, including: '1. Working with elders by building on past strengths; 2. Encouraging the middle-aged and the young-old to prepare for old age by thoughtful anticipation; and 3. Promoting intergenerational interaction for the psychosocial benefit of the old and not-yet-old.'

Vaillant (1993: 151) suggests that the change of focus involved in post-generative age-stages can be conceived of as a shift from 'taking care of one's children to preserving one's culture'. This view introduces a special task for later life, but also fails to solve the core predicament of authentic subjectivity. Preserving culture is seen as a more abstract, sublimated means of caring and as a way of passing accumulated knowledge on to the next generation. Thus, whereas the twin anxieties of preceding adult stages centre on 'How can I commit myself to one person and one job without sacrificing autonomy?' . . . 'Older adults, having safely mastered these tasks, may, as mentors watch this struggle with the same benevolent familiarity with which young adults watch their children' (Vaillant 1993: 146). This shift also fulfils the function of investing in forms of meaning that will outlive the self (Kotre 1984) and the insurance of individual immortality through the direction of others. Alexander *et al.* (1992) consider this to be a particularly individualistic interpretation of passing experience on to succeeding generations which owes much to the priorities of western capitalism.

Generativity and authenticity

As both the conflicts and resolutions of adolescence and old age appear to hinge on life tasks of adulthood, it is worth examining the nature of this central stage in more detail.

At the end of Erikson's summary of his eighth and final stage, one finds this rather curious statement: 'having now reviewed the end of the lifecycle as much as my context permitted, I do feel the urgency to enlarge on a "real" stage – that is, one that mediates between two stages of life – and of the generational cycle itself' (Erikson 1982: 66). He is referring here to the preceding stage, 'generativity', which looks forwards as well as backwards and is concerned with production and reproduction.

Generativity, according to Erikson (1982: 67), expresses the 'spirit of adulthood', which consists of 'the maintenance of the world'. The virtue of this period is care, 'a widening commitment to *take care of* the persons, the products, and the ideas one has learned *to care for*' (italics in original). It encompasses, 'procreativity, productivity and creativity'. McAdams (1988: 276) refers to generativity as 'An action outline for the future which specifies what an individual plans to do in order to leave a legacy of self to the next generation.' This takes place in two steps, namely creating a product and caring for that product. McAdams is most interested in the development of a life story or narrative that can sustain identity and, in this context, procreation and care suggest an extension of self and then a giving up, a recognition of autonomy in the other which makes it simultaneously self and not self. The result becomes a 'life justifying legacy' (McAdams 1985: 276). Thus, a closer reading of generativity itself suggests that the focus of this lifecourse activity is to contribute to what has been called above the 'generational cycle'. Generativity itself is important, in other words, because of the children.

As such, ego psychology resembles disengagement theory (Cumming and Henry 1961) insofar as the subjectivity of personal ageing becomes displaced by a growing focus on self in relation to family, plus an absence of other supportive role options. In both cases the progressive marginality of an ageing identity is cloaked in the guise of its functional value for wider social interests.

It is becoming clear, then, that while generativity rests at the heart of ego psychology, it is also difficult to find an authentic adult subjectivity inside it. While generativity is seen as the central task of mature adulthood, it tells us little about the intrinsic experience of self. Rather, the focus of generativity is again outside the stage itself and concerns the care of others, at other stages. Most notable of these other stages are those of childhood, the function of a mature adult identity being to create the optimal circumstances for successful reproduction of the next generation. Thus other tasks associated with adulthood, such as work and stability in relationships, feed in to this primary organizing principle. This leaves us with the Eriksonian lifecourse as a sort of continuing cycle, without a personally intrinsic centre, for just as childhood is seen as a series of challenges that must be negotiated to become a functional adult, adulthood is seen as a period devoted to creating the conditions for the

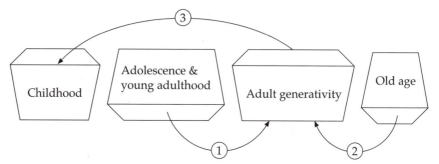

1 Adolescence and young adulthood as preparation for adult generativity.
2 Old age as depending on foundations laid in generativity.
3 Adult generativity aimed at reproducing next generation.

Figure 2.1 Erikson's adult life stages as Chinese boxes.

child's integration into society. As the wrappings of an Eriksonian lifecourse unravel, it appears, then, as a series of Chinese boxes. Each stage, at least in mid and late adulthood, is essentially empty of meaning except insofar as it contains another (see Figure 2.1). And the most problematic of these boxes is the one labelled 'old age', because it is unclear how an authentic role can be found at the end of the lifecourse. Just as you think you've got to that most important, generative, box, you find yourself back at the beginning again.

This problem, 'the problem of the Chinese boxes', highlights a pivotal difference between childhood stages and those of adulthood as conceived in this form of theorizing. Adolescence, it appears, does not simply signify the challenge of developing a stable adult identity, but also marks a qualitative difference in the nature of the bipolar conflicts contained within the stages that precede it and those that follow it. It contains, in other words, a conceptual transition within Erikson's theorizing as well as a practical transition in identity. Childhood priorities, including the development of trust, autonomy, initiative and industry, while they rely upon external conditions, are theorized as intrinsic to the developing psyche. They tell us about the subjective experience of each stage as a form of personal development which is aimed at the self, rather than the development of others. As such they tell us about the experiential reality of childhood for its own sake. This is not the case for generativity and beyond, whose focus, in this sense, is not centred on existential questions of personal development because the key source of fulfilment exists outside the self. The development of others has become the dominant factor in determining any insight the model might give into adult subjectivity. Other aspects are eclipsed except insofar as they can subsist within that age-stage framework. Another way of putting this is to imagine the practical implications of the conceptual model were they to be applied to a therapeutic context. Up until adolescence, an Eriksonian therapist might take a keen interest in you, your experience and mastery of the world, but after adolescence there is a sudden shift: he or she no longer seems interested in you, only in how successful you are in bringing up the kids and contributing to your workplace. Prior to that age the theory tells a story based on an authentic exploration of self; after it, it does not.

Thus the Eriksonian perspective is, at the core of its theoretical reasoning, child-centred, and tells us little about the cultivation of self in the mature imagination. This is so much the case that even the elders interviewed in *Vital Involvement in Old Age* turn out to be the parents of children interviewed in the original longitudinal study (Erikson *et al.* 1986: 21). This observation in itself suggests an alternative explanation to why Erikson *et al.*'s (1986) interviewees did not remember the trials and crises noted in the original longitudinal study. The problems were those of their children's development rather than their own.

This child centredness differs from that of classical Freudianism. For Freud, the prime concern was to allow adults to shake off problems arising from childhood, thus containing the tendency to see the internal workings of the mind as dominated by conflicts arising from early development. For Erikson, the primary focus of adulthood would be to raise the next generation, and our understanding of the adult psyche is only seriously examined insofar as it contributes to that objective. This is what one might expect from a man who undertook his own analysis with Anna Freud, a founder of child and family psychotherapy and whose own generative age-stage concerned the relationship between childhood and society. Viewed in this light, it is unsurprising that Erikson's schema focuses predominantly on the early years of life, with only two from eight stages referring to mature adulthood (Jacobs 1986). The surprise, perhaps, is that he has been heralded so widely as a champion of later life development, presumably because of a dearth of alternatives at the time.

Ego psychology and Fordism

Whilst ego psychology does not appear to see childhood as formative in the Freudian sense, its reliance on generativity as a source of adult coherence places child-rearing as the core task for a mature imagination. There is a social conformity hiding within the commonsensual 'obviousness' of the age-stage model. The age-stage approach has been criticized by Buss (1979) and Andrews (1991) as being too individualistic and as failing to recognize social and cultural influences on development. It is also possible to argue that the core failure of age-staging consists of its inability to step beyond the social context in which it is embedded. It is, in other words, so influenced by social structures as never to get beyond them.

For Erikson (1982: 90), the embedding nature of social structure lends that necessary coherence to the lifecourse as it 'lifts the known facts into a context apt to make us realise their nature'. This results in an uncritical relation to that context, which has been exacerbated by the subsequent work of Vaillant (1993) and Kivnick (1993), which has drained earlier explorations of ego psychology of its conflictual tensions and problematic.

In retrospect it is possible to see, within the eight stages of development, a 'Fordist' or production line model of the lifecourse, closely related to the needs of contemporary capital at the time that Erikson and others were generating their theoretical ideas. If the fulcrum of the lifecourse can be found in the generation of a stable career and family, then just as one's ability to produce and reproduce accrues value under capitalism, a successful lifecourse positions childhood and later life as a preparation for and hangover from the 'real business' of making things and people in the material world. Unfortunately, as Lynott and Lynott (1996) have pointed out, this historical period was also marked by implicit theorizing, based on a belief that truths about human development were increasingly being discovered and that universal patterns of ageing identity were being observed independently of socio-historical context. Thus, rather than stages being seen as one possible way of conceptualizing the lifecourse, they were perceived as the one and only way. The result was a preoccupation with function, adjustment and fit of lifestyle to the demands of contemporary production. An example of this in Erikson's own research can be seen in the degree to which cohort effects are taken as normative. In *Vital Involvement in Old Age*, 29 elders were interviewed, from the same cohort as the Eriksons themselves. This is presented as a positive advantage by the investigators, insofar as it increases empathy and mutual understanding. However, its disadvantage, that it obscures the identification of shared assumptive realities, is not explored. Both the functional approach adopted and cohort specificity mean that investigators might not recognize change, or might minimize its impact if a predetermined life cycle itself minimizes crises and obscures alternatives. By the symbolic ordering of events being handed over to society, the possibility of legitimate construction of other personal narratives is lost.

Schroots (1996: 744) has indicated that stage theories have difficulty in accommodating an increase in psycho-social variability that occurs with age because 'The developmental tasks of an infant are relatively universal, but the tasks in later life are dependent as much on personal experiences as on general principles.' Thus, the older the stage, the greater the psycho-social diversity. A stage-based model, with fixed and functional definitions of appropriate development, would, according to this argument, become increasingly unable to contain the variety of experience that maturity and later life have accrued. This is another way of saying that stage-based models with fixed characteristics become increasingly inappropriate with age, especially if they are premised on a limited and conformist vision of what late life might hold.

The value of ego psychology for the mature imagination

So where does this analysis of the Eriksonian life cycle leave us in terms of the positioning of mature and late adulthood? It can now be seen that while a move towards ego-functioning avoids some of the conceptual problems inherent in classical psychoanalysis, it has created new difficulties for the understanding of self and identity in midlife and beyond and reshaped some old ones. The much anticipated focus on adult development that was promised by ego psychology seems on second inspection to be essentially hollow. Again the question turns on the centrality of childhood and the uncritical acceptance of contemporary social stereotypes of adult ageing. The deep structure of the approach is child-centred in a number of respects. Most notably, a critical analysis of the internal structure of the position indicates that adult stages not only draw their primary meaning from earlier stages, they cease to achieve independent existential priorities. Further, qualitative differences between childhood stages of development and adult ones subtly privilege the former. It is not so much that childhood is seen as formative in this model, rather that it is presented as more interesting and valuable. At each stage, however, the conflicts and priorities approach descriptions of socially accepted milestones, each of which contains a right and wrong direction. This is not simply a chronological contingency, but a contingency of meaning and experience. Erikson's real creativity lies in what he has to say about psychological development concerning social expectation and child-rearing. There is a stark absence of interest in a subjectivity of adulthood.

The positioning of mature adulthood emerging from ego psychology is very much of a second-hand existence. Generativity emerges as core to adult identity and at the centre of this one finds procreation. Later life relies on prior good planning and an interest in handing on to younger generations. Inner directed growth of the adult psyche is not subject to significant conceptual elaboration; instead followers of Erikson have increased an emphasis on coherence, and an uncritical elaboration of social conformity.

Whereas it has been argued that King's (1974, 1980) debate within psychoanalysis achieved an unpeeling of subjective and social attributes associated with chronological age, Erikson and his followers have been busy restitching consciousness and the social order. What becomes apparent is the centrality of generativity as the fulcrum of the human lifecourse. However, while the adult lifecourse would appear to depend on generativity, this is itself contingent upon reproduction and conformity to economic productive processes. If adolescence marks the entry into an enduring adult identity, mid-adulthood marks its fruition in production and reproduction and, most notably, the creation of the next generation. The integrity of old age is doubly disadvantaged within this system. First, as a final stage, it can look only back and not forwards within the constraints of the model. Second, successful negotiation of this final stage is seen as contingent both on previous planning at other stages and on being able to contribute vicariously to the tasks allotted to those preceding stages. One therefore needs to look elsewhere for the germ of a critical adult psychology.

JUNG AND ANALYTICAL PSYCHOLOGY

If Erikson's response to an underdeveloped psychodynamic theorizing of maturity was to create a system that tied adaptive development to social expectation, Jung travelled in the opposite direction. Where Erikson and his followers have explored the relationship between the ego and the social world such that fantasy activity is almost entirely eclipsed, Jung's analytical psychology looked for meaning in an increasingly close relationship between the ego and an inner world of the imagination. Where ego psychology positioned later life as a period of second-hand fulfilments and functions, analytical psychology suggested that the aims and objectives of mature adulthood had little in common with those of earlier adult life at all. Whereas Erikson can be seen as developing aspects of psychoanalysis in a linear progression from Anna and Sigmund Freud, Jung's intellectual development is marked by a fundamental split from the founding discipline.

From psychoanalysis to an analysis of adulthood

When Jung and Freud argued about the nature of therapy and the interpretation of previously unconscious material, the break was irreparable (McGuire 1991). It heralded a period of turmoil and acrimonious debate which eventually resulted in the development of analytical psychology, as Jung came to call his own version of psychotherapy and its accompanying theoretical position. As part of this reformulation Jung explored a number of ideas that have made analytic psychology a far more receptive framework for the examination of issues in mature adulthood.

First, Jung found it necessary to formulate his own dissatisfactions with the psychoanalytic model, which he found both restrictive and reductive. It was restrictive insofar as it contained a model of the psyche that had become something of an article of faith in terms of structure and the primacy of sexuality. It was reductive insofar as the formative influences on adult identity had been reduced to the resolution of oedipal conflicts in childhood. Second, as part of the break with Freud, which occurred during 1912 and 1913, Jung lost his own analyst. Without Freud to guide him, Jung was forced to engage in self-analysis and developed what he later called the process of active imagination. Third, movement beyond the theoretical strait-jacket of mainstream psychoanalysis and the development of his own methodology allowed Jung to formulate a new model of the psyche that began to address the workings of adult psychology in itself and within its own terms of reference.

Jung's dissatisfaction with the psychoanalytic model can be seen in his essay *The Transcendent Function*, written in 1916. As Homans (1995) has pointed out, Jung's view was that in an initial period of psychotherapy, things progressed very much as Freud would have predicted. Transference relationships were formed around parental role relationships, which could, if therapy were successful, be used to rework dysfunctional solutions set originally in childhood. Thus dreams and other phenomena originating from the unconscious could be accurately seen as giving shape to libidinal energy, itself based on childhood sexuality and the personal route taken to oedipal resolution. However, Jung maintained that while psychoanalysis helps to clear away the unfinished business of childhood, it has nothing to say about what happens next. The adult is thought to be cured and that is that.

The inadequacy of psychoanalysis stemmed from its silence on how to interpret the new situations and possibilities made available by the removal of these childhood problems and the resulting release of psychological energy that had previously been repressed. 'The continued application of Freudian techniques does not help in this new situation, for the patient has already assimilated the contents of these interpretations . . . hence a new conceptual framework is required to account for this process' (Homans 1995: 97). According to Homans, this realization created a turning point in analytical psychology that resulted in a new understanding of transference and a distinction being made between a personal unconscious, containing memories from an individual's own history, and collective patterns within the psyche, such as archetypal images that depend on universal forms of human experience. It also contributed to a new formulation of the adult lifecourse which could now be thought of as consisting of first and second halves of life.

First and second halves of adult life

In Jung's new formulation, the first half of life, which spans early adulthood up to middle age, consists of a period in which identity is consolidated

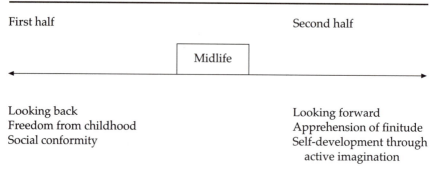

First half   Second half

Midlife

Looking back   Looking forward
Freedom from childhood   Apprehension of finitude
Social conformity   Self-development through
                                         active imagination

Figure 2.2 Jungian 'halves of adult life'.

around the personal will, and as part of this process the constraints of childhood need to be cast aside. It is thus 'Enough to clear away all the obstacles that hinder expansion and ascent' (Jung 1967d: 114), the object of which is to 'win for oneself a place in society and to transform one's nature so that it is more or less fitted in to this kind of existence' (Jung 1967d: 771). The kind of existence that is being referred to concerns the adaptation of the inner world of the younger adult to the demands of her or his social environment. Thus, while the first half of life feels as if it is a period of increasing freedom from the personal past, it is, in reality, running to embrace the snares of social conformity. Of course, Jung is having a little dig at Freud here, as traditional psychoanalysis has now itself been reduced to the technology of social control. Psychoanalysis thereby fails to transcend and ultimately results in the restoration of a social persona. By contrast, the task of the second half of life, and for Jung this represented a road to authentic self-knowledge, was to 'divest the self of the false wrappings of the persona on the one hand, and the suggestive power of primordial images on the other' (Jung 1967b: 269).

A need for social achievement and acceptance during the first half of life is replaced by a desire for personal coherence and completeness in the second. When compared to Freudian analytic theory, analytic psychology was, Jung claimed, allied to a constructive as opposed to a reductive view of adult development, and one which pointed towards the future rather than looking back to the personal past. It therefore developed beyond the clearing away of persistent infantile desires towards the assimilation of wider elements of the unconscious. As one ceases to look over one's shoulder at past constraints, attention is also drawn to the limits to future existence, as death becomes an increasingly important point of personal reference (see Figure 2.2).

The core task of this second half of life concerns what Jung called individuation. Individuation has been described by Samuels *et al.* (1986) as the process by which persons become themselves, 'whole, indivisible and distinct from others', and results in successively greater territories of the self becoming amenable to consciousness. Thus 'a person in the second half of life . . . no longer needs to educate his conscious will, but . . . to understand the meaning of his individual life, needs to experience his own inner being. Social usefulness is no longer an aim for him, although he does not deny its desirability . . . increasingly, too, this activity frees him from morbid dependence, and he thus acquires an inner stability and new trust in himself' (Jung 1967e: 110). The process of individuation is seen as naturally occurring in the second half of life, and 'the transformation processes which make the transition possible have long been prepared in the unconscious and are only waiting to be released' (Jung 1933a: 528).

Awareness of a change in life priorities is thought to begin between the ages of 35 and 40, although chronological ages are only approximate as Jung saw the unconscious as relatively autonomous, with a life of its own and a time scale that 'will out'. From this perspective 'separating and objectifying the unconscious is essentially a process of maturity' and an 'Active imagination is the germ material of later life' (Weaver 1973: 11).

Thus, according to the Jungian model, first and second halves of adult life contain markedly different existential goals, which provide the spadework for an authentic subjectivity for mature adulthood. Further, discussion of the adult lifecourse has been separated from issues of illness and cure, and in reading Jung, one is given a series of signposts towards what a general subjectivity of maturity might look like. The tasks associated with this second period involve the discovery of parts of the self that had been repressed during the first half's search for conformity, an increased sensitivity to an inner life beyond the limits of the personal will and a looking forward, induced, in part, by an increasing awareness of finitude and mortality (Biggs 1993a).

'Getting stuck' and the active imagination

It is clear from Jung's writings that he did not simply develop a new typology for adult development, but also found that new therapeutic methods were required when addressing mid- and late-life development. Unlike the situation in psychoanalysis, there is considerable evidence that the founder of analytical psychology had significant experience of working with mature adults, the majority of whom were women. In *The Aims of Psychotherapy* (1931: 83), for example, Jung states that 'About a third of my cases are not suffering from any clinically definable neurosis, but from the senselessness and aimlessness of their lives . . . Fully two thirds of my patients are in the second half of life.'

The problems brought by mature patients are more often than not referred to as 'getting stuck', as the priorities of the first half of life cease to provide meaning. Jung recommended abandoning the strictures of psychoanalysis in favour of a non-directive and open-ended approach to this problem. 'I resolved for the present not to bring any theoretical premises to bear upon them, but to wait and see what they would tell of their own accord. My aim became to leave things to chance' (Jung 1961: 170). The ultimate aim of psychoanalysis was to ensure that patients are freed to continue to use the unconscious in their everyday lives, rather than being driven by it. The object of this new method was to enhance a process of increased individuation, which was thought to occur naturally in maturity, when circumstances allowed.

The method suggested by analytic psychology has come to be called 'active imagination'. Chodorow (1997) suggests that Jung began to experiment with active imagination, between 1913 and 1916, as a 'middle-aged man in crisis', although he did not publish his findings until much later (1935). For Jung, the great benefit of active imagination was that it enabled the distinguishing of oneself from the unconscious contents of the imagination. This he contrasted with the experience of dreams, in which the imagination passively received communications from the unconscious such that the dreaming subject was totally immersed in the dream world. Just as in everyday life an absence of awareness of unconscious influences can lead to the acting out of their dynamic, so dreaming failed to allow the dreamer to recognize that he or she was dreaming. The object of active imagination was to separate out the conscious ego from the imaginative material in order to achieve a dialogue between the two. Thus, 'A product is created which is influenced by both conscious and unconscious, embodying the striving of the unconscious for light and the striving of the conscious for substance' (Jung 1916: 168).

Chorodow (1997: 10) identifies two stages in the development of an active imagination: 'First letting the unconscious come up and second, coming to terms with the unconscious . . . it is a natural sequence that might go on over many years.' The first step simply consists of letting things happen, a sort of meditative daydream in which material is allowed to emerge and can be consciously observed. 'At first the unconscious takes the lead while the conscious ego serves as a kind of attentive inner witness.' Then, 'in the second part of active imagination consciousness takes the lead. As the affects and images of the unconscious flow into awareness, the ego enters actively into the experience. This part might begin with a spontaneous string of insights; the larger task of evaluation and integration remains. Insight must be converted into an ethical obligation – to live it in life' (*ibid.*).

The active imagination thus involves fantasy activity that includes the participation of the conscious ego. The ego can thereby enter into remembered communication with the contents of the unconscious and become an active player in the narrative as it develops. The psyche is here seen as being an autonomous realm with which the ego cooperates, rather than territory that must be conquered. The focus shifts from the sovereignty of the ego to a development of inner relationships. And the response to an emerging subjectivity of mature adulthood is to make available the tools of self-exploration to older adults.

Weaver (1973) links active imagination to the development of a 'personal myth' around which inner and outer realities can be restructured. However, according to the Jungian tradition, one can be seduced by personal myth so that the myth takes over and is living you rather than you it. Active imagination allows a dialogue to take place between the self and these mythic images, which, in the mind's eye, can take human form. It 'makes it possible to have a discussion with them without the ego being swamped by them in a way in which they are indistinguishable from one's thoughts and moods' (Weaver 1973: 7). Indeed, an active imagination would seem to suggest two forms of consciousness, which in another setting have been examined by Brennan (1997). The first form of consciousness consists of the instrumental awareness associated with the psychoanalytic ego, 'a repository of received views, planning in advance and one form of intentionality' (Brennan 1997: 91–2). However, Brennan also hypothesizes a second form, a 'life-force' which is mindful rather than driven and a source of intuitive creativity. This second form exists beyond language and beneath everyday activity, and involves a suspension of the ego-control which 'coincides with rejuvenation'.

The autonomy attributed to fantasy activity in analytical psychology, that it is literally seen to have a life of its own, also has a bearing on the representation of age-based identities within the psyche. Rather than being interpreted primarily in terms of transference relationships, here associations and fantasy figures become archetypal figures that contain special (yet also universal) properties. They become messengers from the unconscious. The developmental characteristics of these archetypal figures has been elaborated elsewhere (Biggs 1989, 1993a), and of particular interest to the study of mature identity formation are the wise old woman (Weaver 1973) and man (Middelcoop 1985). While 'wise elders' inevitably come to reflect cultural stereotypes in some of their attributes, their main function in the adult psyche is liminal. That is to say, they are gatekeepers who indicate an alternative state of being, partly by their reminding presence as persons in later life, and partly as a guide to a state of affairs that the active subject has not experienced to date. Resistance to the influence of wise elders would be a response to their role as harbingers of personal change as much as it is to the properties of old age itself. By nurturing skills of active imagination, the possibility emerges of entering into dialogue with elders who inhabit one's inner world, or indeed an internal dialogue between different age-specific representations of the self. The bearing this has on intergenerational communication is twofold. First, Samuels (1985) has argued that all archetypal figures are filled out by reference to culture and personal experience, which suggests that an increased dialogue may influence relations in external 'reality'. Second, Hillman (1970) has developed an archetypal psychology in which responses to external objects (which include people) are mediated by the internal archetypal matrix of images. In other words, one would respond to an older person, child, woman, man as a reflection of these internal characters as well as individuals with their own personal identities. Both of these positions would indicate a close relationship between the character of images from the imagination and relations between individuals and groups in the external, social world. Modifications in the psychological arena would have a reciprocal effect on actual relations between generations.

Drawing on Jungian ideas, Tornstam (1996) has identified the psychology of later life as concerning the task of 'gerotranscendence'. This, he proposes, can be qualitatively distinguished from Erikson's 'ego-integrity' and forms of disengagement in that it includes elements of both. 'A high degree of gerotranscendence is related to higher degrees of both social activity and life satisfaction simultaneously as the degree of social activity becomes less important in attaining satisfaction' (Tornstam 1996: 38). Later life, can, according to this perspective, be connected with both social activity and solitary 'philosophizing'. Tornstam (1994) collected experiences of Swedish (52–97 years) and Danish (74–100) older adults, and indicates that while external losses increase in later life, there is an absence of reported loneliness. He suggests that adults approach identity 'more like a Buddhist' as they age, which he interprets as an intrinsic drive towards transcendence marked by 'positive solitude' and an increased broad-mindedness. This is complemented by an enhanced awareness of the difference between self and role, in the sense of distinguishing between the development of what is unique about the self rather than conforming to an appropriate social niche. Such processes are connected to more active and complex coping patterns in social situations. Schroots (1996) notes that gerotranscendence refers to active multi-coping strategies rather than the defensiveness and social breakdown implied by disengagement. These elaborations of Jungian themes highlight the creativity and flexibility that can occur as a correlate of increased inner-directedness in later life.

The Jungian inheritance

Jung leaves us with an understanding of the subjectivity of mature adulthood that is very different from both psychoanalysis and ego psychology. In many respects it is as if other orthodoxies have been stood on their heads. Rather than seeing mature adulthood as a period in which self-exploration becomes increasingly difficult, analytical psychology makes a virtue out of individuation. The mature imagination is described as consisting of increased insight and inner-directedness. This is no period of vicarious existence, but one in which the mature adult is seen as having a duty to attend to the self; indeed, interpersonal relations are rarely touched on. By comparison with the Eriksonian life cycle, the Jungian model results in a critical stance towards social mores. The first half of life is thought to lead to a diminution of the personality precisely because of younger adult concerns about achievement within an established social order. From a Jungian standpoint, ego psychology appears to consist of a 'history of social personas', persona being theorized as a superficial and essentially dysfunctional means of social adaptation. It is partly this cynicism concerning social influences on the psyche, and a tendency to introversion in the personality of Jung himself, that leads to the positioning of later life as a period of personal growth involving a considerable amount of inward attention.

As the second half of life is thought of as being quite different from the first in terms of existential priorities, an examination of the subjectivity of this second phase is sharply differentiated from childhood. Childhood is viewed neither as a source of adult problems nor as a formative and central focus of the lifecourse as a whole. Indeed, it is hardly mentioned, except as a repository of issues that need to be cleared up before the real business of adult development can get under way.

It is also apparent that the properties that this model associates with midlife and old age are seen as part of a natural maturational process which can be enhanced by therapeutic intervention, but is by no means dependent upon it. The non-directive application of active imagination allows a diversity of experience to be recognized and given voice in mature adulthood. While King (1973) has contributed to the understanding of transference phenomena in later life, analytical psychology has expanded our understanding of how figures from the inner world represent age and ageing. Both these trends, one emphasizing interpersonal perception and the other intrapersonal symbolization, contribute to the disaggregation of chronology and social norms from the the inner experience of age. Ageing emerges as a process of increasing multiplicity and dialogue, which, perhaps paradoxically, engenders an increasingly intact and rounded sense of self.

Mature adulthood is thus seen as being a time of natural expansion for the self, in contrast to the constraining presence of social expectation. This arguably results in an overly optimistic conceptualization of later life, which pays insufficient attention to the effects of bodily ageing or structured inequalities within an ageing population. However, the advantages of this perspective, both as a personal narrative and as a cultural understanding of later life, are considerable. The story, from midlife onwards, includes the possibility of personal development that is unique to this life phase, and invites caution as to the advisability of plotting a course based on priorities from other parts of the lifecourse.

3

Postmodern ageing

MODERNITY AND POSTMODERNITY

In addition to the psychodynamic debate on ageing identity, there has also been a growing acknowledgement that the social circumstances in which identities are played out may be shifting dramatically. Attention has shifted towards the surface manifestations of identity rather than deeper structuration. These changes have been characterized as a movement away from conditions of modernity to something else, which has been called variously late capitalism (Jameson 1984), high modernity (Giddens 1991) or postmodernity (Featherstone 1991). Whereas the guiding principles of modernity could be thought of as a belief in linear progress, technical expertise and universal explanations of human behaviour, these new developments are marked by a suspicion that progress from one perspective might mean calamity from another, an awareness of diversity that verges on fragmentation and a sense that riskiness and uncertainty pervade social life.

This state of affairs might be more realistically thought of as an intensification of processes that have been developing since the Western Enlightenment and the growth of industrial societies worldwide. It has been argued that as the world moves faster and faster, and gets increasingly complex, so the roots of personal identity become stressed and insecure. These circumstances necessitate strategies which are adapted to change, one aspect of which is a movement of interest away from static content to the importance of process in the maintenance of an adult identity. Not so much what individuals think they are, then, as how they keep that idea of themselves going. Models of ageing and of personal change which have emphasized defined age characteristics may now be seen as attempts to stabilize ageing identities against an increasingly chaotic background.

Indeed, some writers consider that change and the impact of consumer culture are sufficiently intense to dislocate behaviours and attributes from their established meanings altogether. In the centrifuge of contemporary society, it is proposed that identities become detached and recombined in ways that may have no relation to their original meaning and context. Whereas modernist thinking has tended to emphasize the threats that rapid social change holds for personal identity, postmodernism evidences a tendency towards a celebration of the multiplicity and recombinations that can result. Qualities that have traditionally been associated with age, for example, would no longer be fixed, and older adults may be able to create new forms of self-presentation (Gilleard 1996). The promise, as far as ageing and identity are concerned, is that one might somehow choose not to become old.

MODERNITY AND UNCERTAINTY

The contradictory nature of modern existence is still best summed up by Marx and Engel's (1888) observation that contemporary society cannot survive without constantly revolutionizing its productive base, on which human relationships depend. This process is experienced as one in which 'All fixed, fast-frozen relations, with their train of ancient and venerable prejudices and opinions are swept away, all new-formed ones become antiquated before they can ossify. All that is solid melts into air, all that is holy is profaned, and man is at last compelled to face with sober senses, his real conditions of life' (Marx and Engels 1888: 83).

This quote eloquently conveys the tremendous energy within modern society and suggests a number of core points about the modern human condition. First, the self is surrounded by constant change, brought about by competition to make ever cheaper and more effective goods. Second, the most important, and defining, scenario for identity is that of work, as a relationship of production in which value is conferred and change made possible. It is, in other words, one's position in relation to production that defines identity and social consciousness. Further, pre-existing anchors for identity are fast being eroded, which will eventually confront human beings with the underlying dynamic that structures their relationships one to another other. For Marx, these hidden relations were based on class antagonism and it was a class identity, an identity based on economics, that was constantly being obscured. Because the system was in a continual state of flux, however, attempts would be made by powerful groups to fix social relations and how these relationships were seen. Dominant and progressive groups would contest this territory, and eventually this form of progress would give birth to a future in which contemporary contradictions are resolved.

Late life, as political economists such as Estes (1979), Townsend (1986), Walker (1986) and Phillipson and Walker (1986) have observed, does not fare well under this regime. Adult ageing is increasingly marginalized with regard to work. The spaces made available, especially to older adults, are structured in terms of dependency, and they are commonly perceived as a burden on more productive parts of society. Rather than their life experience being valued, it is construed as obsolescent in the headlong rush towards a better future.

Age, ageing, maturity and late life are all identities that are affected by these conditions and by the remedies that are made available. These are effects that go further than the traditional image of older people failing to keep up with dizzying change. There are biases at a more abstract level, including the privileging of the future over the past and the importance of work as an organizing principle which is itself age-stratified, working to place mature adulthood at a disadvantage. However, there are also trends, suggested by Giddens (1991) among others, that point to certain advantages over the negative attribution of age. If identities can indeed be recreated without significant reference to where they have traditionally been embedded, might this not also open up the possibility of mature identities disconnected from stereotyping and over-determination?

Psychologically speaking, modernity is both frightening and exciting. It is a setting in which, according to Frosh (1991: 11–12), 'human relationships are possible, but are always being undercut and destroyed. An environment in which personal integrity means something as a potentiality, but is always in danger of being fragmented by forces beyond our control.' One must sift through the contradictory experiences of modern life to find an enduring sense of self. Once discovered, the self is always in danger of erosion and in need of regeneration. What distinguishes modern consciousness from that of other eras is an unsettling demand that it takes both itself and the period in which it exists as an object of constant interrogation and renewal (Venn 1997). Modernity is characterized, then, as both undercutting the status quo and a source of increasing interconnection, which Giddens (1991) identifies with a progressive disembedding from traditional structures that might contextualize and structure the lifecourse. Accordingly, social relations are freed from the hold of specific positions, such as age-stages, and can simultaneously be recombined 'across wide time–space distances'. Castoriades (1997) has suggested that contemporary capitalism holds out the promise of creative autonomy, plus the threat of external control, and this contradiction goes some way to describe the shape identity takes under modern conditions. It produces certainty, in particular and restricted forms, plus the threat of vertiginal uncertainty. Modernity can, then, be seen as giving rise to a narrative of a core self, beset by difficulties and assaults to its integrity, that is *kept* stable over time. The past is a critical reference point in the search for a better future state. In order to maintain its integrity, the self must divine strategies that accommodate a continual state of becoming. Identity, just like the forces of production, is in need of continuous servicing, in order to maintain a balance between determinacy and indeterminacy and ensure its survival.

This description of the modern self speaks a language that is recognizable to the psychodynamic project. They are related enterprises that emphasize progress, the hidden nature of truth and the importance of creating an authentic narrative. The psychotherapies protect identity against being crushed by this juggernaut, and teach us how to make the most of what personal indeterminacy can be found. A belief in the possibility of self-development is thereby sustained, even in the face of the brutalities of modernization. Psychotherapy constitutes a search for continuity in an unstable and uncertain world, so that we can, in Berman's (1982) phrase, keep on keeping on. Psychoanalysis is modern in the sense that it is committed to the uncovering of 'deep' structures that will increase the circumference of personal control, contained within a meta-narrative that explains the superiority of the present over the past. This is embodied in the struggle to make sense of and overcome irrational psychological drives, and also in the suggestion that social cohesion is achieved at considerable psychic cost and suffering. The relationship between the person and society is therefore problematic.

THE POSTMODERNIZATION OF PSYCHOTHERAPY

Multiplying ageing identity

The psychotherapies form an important source of information about legitimized characteristics of the maturing adult. They also tell us something about the process of identity management, the techniques used to maintain and repair the self, over and above the attributes that any identity might contain. Changes in technique are also part and parcel of new understandings of how the self can be sustained in everyday life. The tactics and strategies we use to keep our identities going on a daily basis will tend both to reflect the technologies of contemporary psychotherapy and to influence them as part of a rich, but often tacit, cultural dialogue on adult identity.

Frosh (1991) points out that while Freud's patients were suffering from too much repression, they were not mad. Rather, in the restrictive circumstances of turn-of-the-century Vienna, 'their toleration of the demands of society required renunciation of certain inner demands . . . Which if acted on would lead to the devastation of their social relationships' (Frosh 1991: 34). Freud's great invention was to find a way to recalibrate their psychic processes and, in so doing, to render them more able in the struggle to maintain order in the face of internal chaos. So, while psychoanalysis radically destabilized thinking on the human condition, its goal was to integrate individuals back into society. 'I offer you no consolation,' says Freud at the beginning of *Civilization and Its Discontents* (1930). There is no escape from the filling out of a social blueprint because the alternative would be the chaotic, the irrational and the destructive in the human soul. Society precludes the possibility of acting out erotic and murderous impulses, and in so doing ensures the survival of the species. The task of adulthood consists, according to this perspective, of a struggle to achieve and maintain a 'working' identity. Not anarchic pleasure and anger, but 'ordinary unhappiness' becomes the order of the adult day.

Erikson's and Jung's theories of adult psychology can be seen, in retrospect, as different instances of closure around this central issue. While Jung saw psychoanalysis as contributing to an overbearing social control, the direction taken by Erikson reflects the view that such theorizing insufficiently connected the self to society. They therefore draw the line around identity and its containing structure in different places. The Eriksonian approach emphasizes balance between different stages the adult passes through towards personal coherence and continuity. There is a preoccupation with binding the sequential elements of the lifecourse together into a meaningful whole. This element of coherence is provided by embedding identity firmly into social structuration, with a clear goal in generativity. Within this model, threats to the self emerge through the unsuccessful negotiation of stability which would otherwise form the basis for the next stage of development. It consists of a domestication of psychoanalysis in which the unconscious hardly makes an appearance, except as a 'striving for continuity of personal character' or 'the silent doings of ego-synthesis'. It is an attempt to fix ageing identities in response to the challenge of modernity.

For Jung, adult coherence centred on a continuing process of individuation. Social structuration, when not seen as irrelevant, was seen as an impediment to the elaboration of an increasing amount of personal material that becomes consciously available. Rather than being bound by 'false wrappings', an antidote to meaningless existence is seen in an entry into dialogue with the unconscious. This model thereby retains some of the terror of unconscious forces and the creativity of the irrational. The Jungian 'lifecourse' is not linear in the sense that age-stages are; rather, it is liminal. Liminality refers to a state of progressive transformation and transition, and has its linguistic root in the concept of a threshold. According to this perspective, the adult psyche is opened to increasing indeterminacy as multiple options present themselves for negotiation. The negotiating, however, contributes to a strengthening of the core self, the increasingly individuated negotiator.

Both, in their different ways, introduce an element of play into the debate on the nature of self, identity and the relationship between the parts and the whole. Separate identities are peeled off from an undifferentiated core and the relationship between age and identity is loosened. Erikson's linear progression suggests that many different parts of the self appear as one progresses through the lifecourse. Thus a multiplicity of age-related identities occurs over time. In analytic psychology's entry into negotiation with the unconscious and the irrational, the parts are organized coexistently and also have age-specified characteristics. A multiplicity of identities is therefore said to exist at the same time within the individual psyche. However, a problem exists for both, because there is a lack of fit between social expectation and experience and, while the solutions suggested by ego and analytical psychologies are radically different, they hold in common the need to keep a core self together and resist disintegration. Erikson and Jung thereby provide different solutions to this abiding problem of the modern adult self.

The modern (and modernist) problem of the ageing self that emerges from these developments can be described as follows. In maturity, the self has both more options and more experience to draw on. It becomes more whole. Whereas, in young adulthood, the life-force acts as a source of driving energy, in mature adulthood it emerges as an organizing principle. However, this expansion of the self occurs within an increasingly hostile and uncertain set of social circumstances. The question arises whether it is possible for the mature adult to keep a coherent core self together in these inhospitable circumstances. Self-identity is both loosened up and subject to restriction aimed at exercising some control over the place of ageing individuals.

'Peeling off' and 'loosening up'

Two trends can be identified from an examination of ageing and identity in this context. The first can be described as a process of 'peeling off'. Peeling off refers to a trend towards the uncoupling of qualities that were previously thought to be integral, to be more or less the same thing. Examples include: the separation of adult ageing and increasing rigidity in the psyche, such that perspectives on maturity include variety and the expansion of previously underdeveloped aspects of the self; distinguishing between chronological age and the internal experience of self so that one's age no longer leads to easy assumptions about how old one feels; and distinguishing between social expectation and personal development, so that certain age-stages are seen to depend upon specific cultural contexts rather than being a universal blueprint that discriminates between successful and unsuccessful ageing.

Second, a process of 'loosening up' is suggested by increased flexibility in the relationship between qualities once they have been distinguished one from another. Examples here would include the proposals that different images of the ageing self exist within the psyche, and can interact with each other or become dominant in particular contexts but not others, or that internal thoughts and feelings can be transferred on to others and in some cases others identify with them. These processes facilitate the adoption of different identities at different times and in different places. Loosening up also refers to a move towards non-directive approaches in counselling and therapy, which encourage the exploration of personal experience, rather than reducing it, through interpretation, to meanings that fit a particular theory of identity at any one point in the lifecourse.

Peeling off and loosening up have contributed to thinking about the lifecourse as containing a variety of shapes or textures. However, it would be wrong to conclude that psychotherapy has rejected the idea that there is a personality or life-force that lends experience coherence and purpose. Rather, these trends contribute to a view of adult ageing as both malleable and maintaining the notion of a core sense of self (McAdams 1997). This self is the someone who is doing the shaping, who performs an identity, and ensures that there is a personal show that is on the road. The shift is qualitative and is reflected in a change of focus from what is said to how it is said, and how it informs what Rustin (1991) has called the 'art of living'. In terms of therapeutic technique, 'practical interest has shifted from developmental history towards the subtleties and ambiguities of the interactions between patient and analyst, on both conscious and unconscious levels' (Rustin 1991: 123). The implications of this change of emphasis for mature adulthood are considerable. In developmental terms, it constitutes a move away from formative events – that this happened in your childhood and caused this to occur now – to a concentration on style and the patterning of contemporary behaviour. The degree to which interpretation is unpeeled from its reliance on early experience would affect the degree to which subjectivities grounded in the experience of adulthood are allowed to emerge. It leads to an interest in intergenerational communication as it happens and the meanings that are created as persons interact with one another. It is, then, a move away from the importance of content and causality to the importance of process and performance and a move with implications for our understanding of lifecourse events.

The influence of psychotherapy is much broader than as a method of individual change: it shapes, and is shaped by, broad notions of personal development in Western societies. It contributes to a modern image of personal identity in a continuous state of 'becoming' and gives it direction. A focus on relationship, the here and now and multiplicity emerge as key to contemporary understandings of identity and change in this context. They represent the form that loosening and peeling off take within contemporary technologies of the self. Each has implications for the positioning of mature adulthood in terms of intergenerational relations, the value attributed to the past and the options for identity that can be legitimately developed.

Relationships

Frosh (1991: 44, 45) has argued that contemporary society has moved 'From the problems of too much depth to those of too much surface', and, in particular, that people now express 'their worries less in terms of self control and more in terms of their inability to form satisfying relationships with others.' This is reflected in a change of emphasis in therapy, from cure through the discovery and exorcizing of past events, to an examination of the dynamic existing between contemporary couples, groups and individuals. The therapist ceases to act as an arbiter of reality because meaning is increasingly understood to be mutually constructed between participants. Stress is placed on the importance of the other as the medium through which the self is experienced and from which feedback is obtained. In terms of technique, the problem for psychotherapy becomes the maintenance of emotional connectedness and therefore, as Rubin (1997: 8) puts it, 'interpretations are tentative, subject to revision with the patient as a partner in their construction.' The analytic task 'is not to discover psychic reality, but to create it'.

A focus on the processes of human relationships increases the use of therapeutic ideas as a guide to everyday, reflexive, living. Giddens (1991: 5), for example, has argued that identities now depend on 'the sustaining of coherent, yet continuously revised, biographical narratives, [that] takes place in the context of multiple choice . . . Reflexively organised life planning, which normally presumes consideration of risks as filtered through contact with expert knowledge, becomes a central feature of the structuring of self-identity.' In other words, the maintenance of a coherent story about the self is no longer a matter of occasional fixing if something goes wrong, but is a continuing process in need of continual 'reskilling'. This is deemed necessary in order to weather transitions that are part and parcel of everyday life. In a similar vein, Kivnick (1993: 23) comments that 'The notion of old age as a time to sit back and reap the psychosocial fruits of earlier efforts must yield to a more realistic view of ongoing, always dynamic re-involvement, reviewing, renewing, reworking.' She reinforces the perception of late life identity as the subject of constant revision and change. However, as part of this incorporation of 'therapy' into the everyday, relationships become increasingly self-contained.

Giddens (1991: 6) refers to this as the development of 'pure relation-ships', 'in which external criteria have become dissolved: the relationship exists solely for whatever rewards the relationship as such can deliver', and trust 'can no longer be anchored in criteria outside the relationship itself.'

Thus, while relationships have come into primary focus, they have also become inward looking, protected from outside frameworks, and take on a life of their own. What goes on within them has, according to this view, become more contingent and less dependent on a single cor-rect notion of conduct, including conduct related to age.

Here and now

A move towards relationship has been paralleled by an increased inter-est in language and dialogue. This has led commentators such as Parker (1996: 447) to suggest that 'psychic processes [have] become located in discourse rather than the self-enclosed interior of individual minds.' The value of this observation stems from an emphasis placed on dialogue itself rather than what it denotes about a personal past. It has, in other words, released identity from history.

The roots of this shift can be seen in an increased importance given to transference phenomena. Transference allows the therapist to concen-trate on the thoughts and feelings that he or she experiences while in the presence of the patient as an important source of information about the patient's own emotional state. Since transference, as a reflection of other relationships, is thought to be enacted in the therapeutic setting, the therapist can heighten the emotional power of an interaction by interpreting the other relationships directly as a part of what is happen-ing between her and the patient. Both of these trends shift the focus of the psychodynamic enterprise away from past or hidden events and towards tacit communications within speech in the here and now. The qualities of relationships that gain emphasis through this process include sustaining an impression of a perpetual present. Parker (1996) points out that contemporary therapy is now concerned with the patterning of discourse and the 'carrying of patterns' in the therapeutic session itself. There has been a change of emphasis. The unconscious is now seen to shape behaviour in the present, and it is possible to read and interpret such patterning without moving beyond the immediate experience of interaction.

This has the advantage of significantly diluting any reduction of adult experience to the residues of childhood contradictions and their attempted solution. And basing adult identity formation in contemporary life contexts provides a powerful set of tools for the discovery of an adult subjectivity.

However, there is also a difficulty in too stringent a focus on here and now events, insofar as it is unclear how continuity and past experience now find a valued space within the new scheme of things. Bollas (1989: 193), for example, observes that 'One of the casualties of the present intense interest in the "here and now" transference interpretation is the diminution of the "there and then".'

The possibility opens for an extreme subjectivity in which the past is simply seen as a metaphor for current concerns and has no point of reference except whatever existential preoccupations are uppermost at any one point in time. 'Recollections' of the past not only serve the selective aims of the present, but cease to have any validity outside of that discourse. Bollas reminds us that there was not only a 'real past' but also 'real memories' of that past, and that it is unclear how a here and now approach can distinguish these historical and personal phenomena from their manipulation or from fantasies in the service of the present. There is a difference, in other words, between narrative and fiction. Privileging the here and now has, in Bollas's (1989: 194) opinion, led to the neglect of 'the need to collect together the detail of a patient's history and to link him to his past in a way that is meaningful.'

When the past is recognized, it appears as source material for current concerns. Thus, Giddens observes, somewhat acerbically, that after divorce individuals are encouraged to 'reach back into [their] early experience and find other images and roots for independence, for being able to live alone and for undertaking the second chances provided' (Giddens 1991: 11). This process is presented as 'the key to reclaiming oneself' by the authors of a self-help manual and contributes to Giddens's theme of identity as increasingly self-referential. It is also important to note that this conception creates a strikingly different relationship with the past from that contained in psychoanalysis. History does not determine the problem and entail freedom from it, but can be used as a ragbag from which the material for a new narrative, more fitting to current circumstances, can be built. The past is not there to be understood, but raw material for immediate concerns.

This argument draws attention to the way that the 'truth' of identity is problematized by this debate. While it is probably the case that we will never be able to know what actually happened to the self or another person, it is a radical departure to assume that all memories simply reflect current story-telling. Rather, memories, as well as being reconstructed, were laid down in particular circumstances and hold those contemporary feelings, interpretations and associations within them. They store, in other words, people's experience of being themselves at that time in their world and it may be valid to retain the authenticity of those original recollections. An emphasis on the here and now, however, only succeeds in including past memory in the service of the present.

Multiplicity and the blurring of boundaries

A third trend in contemporary psychotherapy concerns the possibility that, rather than focusing on the construction of a single personal identity, the psyche includes a variety or multiplicity of options. Elements of this trend can be seen in King's (1980) proposals on transference, Erikson's (1982) sequentially organized life stages and Jung's (1933b) age-related archetypal figures. This loosening of identity has been extended by some writers to suggest that these multiple identities are not simply available, at the same time, in the here and now, but that they should each be credited equal validity. Krippner and Winkler (1995: 277–8), proponents of what has been called consciousness studies, have claimed that a fundamental shift in perspective has occurred 'from one that recognises the value of only a single "normal" state of consciousness to one that values multiple states; from one that sees human development as having a ceiling to one that views such limitations as culturally determined.' According to this position, people can shift from one identity to another, and each of these 'subpersonalities, personal myths, local truths and individual realities' should be seen as equally important.

This disaggregation of the self into many parts also extends to an examination of the connections between individuals, as can be seen in debates over the role of defence mechanisms. The psychodynamic understanding of these mechanisms, including the projection of unpleasant or unwanted thoughts and attributes on to others and projective identification whereby unwanted material from one person is unconsciously accepted by another, suggest an erosion of the boundaries between self and others. Attributes of the personality are spread around by such mechanisms, they appear to exist between people and are maintained by them in ways which render the idea of a psychologically self-contained individual less persuasive. Hinshelwood (1996: 185) suggests, for example, that psychodynamic phenomena such as splitting, projection and introjection, transference and countertransference 'may involve a diffusion of the personality' whereby 'a particular emotion or cognition, sometimes even a mental capacity or function – may become relocated, at least for a while, in the other.'

Accordingly, personal identity may not be as stable and well bounded as has commonly been assumed. Selfhood becomes a horizon, rather than a fixed state, which operates across individual boundaries as well as producing multiple identities. Indeed, under such conditions it becomes increasingly difficult to find a vocabulary that expresses this multiplicity and blurring of boundaries yet maintains the integrity of a core self at all.

Banks (1996) has explored the later life of Virginia Woolf as an example of the inability to achieve Eriksonian integrity under conditions similar to those described above. 'For Woolf, the self is not like a nugget with hard and fast boundaries, but rather, like a cloud with multiple forms, changing components and permeable edges . . . When you met Virginia Woolf on Tuesday you did not see the same woman you had met on Monday' (Banks 1996: 26). She performed selves depending upon whom she was with. So when she reached an age 'when some friends die and others drift away into their own pressing concerns' (Banks 1996: 28), she was left without reliable props with which to maintain such a diffuse patterning of identity. She could not, in other words, reimagine herself as an older woman. Banks proposes that an experience of self as transient and in pieces made it very difficult to come to terms with an integral sense of self, necessary to encounter the challenges and, for Woolf, despair of old age. This description of the experiences that led to Woolf's suicide indicates dangers inherent in multiplicity which lacks props or structures through which an authentic ageing identity can be invented.

In response to these challenges to the task of maintaining an integral self, a psychodynamic understanding would lead one to negotiate chaotic internal and external states, to make sense of them and thereby disarm them. The question would still seem to be how far persons can maintain their selfhood and agency in the face of an increasingly fragmented social world. This point is put rather well by Radden (1996), a social philosopher who, while not working in the psychodynamic tradition, recognizes both the bewildering diversity of everyday life and the possibility of personal continuity. She states that 'Whatever approach we adopt in our explana- tion of divided minds and successive selves, we must acknowledge these unremarkable heterogeneities. Ordinary selves are at best only relatively continuous through time, and at any particular time their unity or oneness is not simple' (Radden 1996: 23). These 'unremarkable heterogeneities of a singular self', she argues, should be treated as a given and a touchstone for contemporary debates on self-identity; and not, by implication, as threaten- ing the existence of an everyday working sense of wholeness. Rather, they indicate a strategy for keeping the self afloat in response to a changing world. Identities can peel off one from another and loosen their relation- ship to a single ordering narrative without losing personal coherence.

CONSUMERISM AND POSTMODERN AGEING

The peeling off and loosening up of the meaning of mature identity, most notable in trends towards relationship, the here and now and multi- plicity, resonates with a broader movement from fixity to flexibility and the idea that identities can be consumed one after another as well as produced by a determining social structure.

If modernist perspectives on the self have tended to rely on production as an organizing principle, contemporary thinking has increasingly looked to patterns of consumption as a basis for diversity and choice in the management of identity. A threat of personal fragmentation is thereby changed into a promise of multiple identity and matching lifestyles. Consumption has increasingly been used as a metaphor for the process of identity maintenance. As part of this process, trends towards 'more surface', such as the loosening of meanings that were previously thought of as fixed and a focus on immediate experience, have led to a rejection of explanations based on depth and time.

Many claims have been made for consumer culture as a phenomenon that marks the management of contemporary identity out from that of preceding historical periods. Crook *et al.* (1992) note, for example, 'the spread of the commodity form into all spheres of life' and point out that the consumption of goods and services has replaced Marx's focus on a relation to production as the principle on which identities are built. And 'at the leading edge of consumerism is a market for ideas about identity offering choice about who one is or might be' (Baddeley 1995: 1075).

So, rather than consumerism being seen as a source of inauthenticity through the manufacture of 'false' needs (Marcuse 1964) and the consumption of ever novel goods as a substitute for genuine self-development (Giddens 1991), it is presented as the raw material of creative identity building. Developments in the mass media and advertising (Williamson 1978; Lury 1996) mediate this process through attempts to make things desirable by association with status, pleasure and lifestyle. This occurs to such an extent, as meanings are grafted on to products that are not intrinsic to them and symbolize attributes beyond their practical function, that symbolic meanings and practical meanings get thoroughly confused. It is then but a short step to begin to detach and recombine meanings in new ways without reference to their original significance. This has led to the proposition that any number of 'floating signifiers' can be used to build an identity, any one of which may be valid under particular conditions. Observation of this position can lead to hyperbolic claims. Featherstone (1983, 1991), for example, notes that an emphasis on lifestyle and consumer culture has led to 'a profusion of information and a proliferation of images which cannot be ultimately stabilised, or hierachised into a system which correlates to fixed social divisions . . . [and] would further suggest the irrelevance of social divisions and ultimately the end of the social as a significant reference point' (Featherstone 1991: 83). A clear implication of this position would be that, given access to consumer culture, social actors can adopt any number of identities that may no longer be directly connected to their material life circumstances. Notions of authenticity and inauthenticity then become meaningless, as any one presentation of self, with the right props, becomes as valid as any other.

Theorizing of this sort can lead from a more restrained view that consumerism provides the resources from which to fashion identity statements, to a strong hypothesis that the notion of a core self is no longer useful in understanding contemporary identity. Selfhood becomes the sum of an arbitrary collection of constructed identities. Munro (1996) suggests that the consumption of identities holds within it a new model for producing the self. Consumer durables become the materials with which the individual creates a 'complex process of prosthesis', a 'labour of self', used to make individuals visible to each other. Munro argues that one cannot, however, see this simply as an extension of a core identity, in other words, as the use of props to decorate something that is itself stable and unchanging. Identity is changed by the process of consumption and therefore is not what it was.

A radical deconstruction of the self is most closely associated with the work of Jean Baudrillard (1990). Extending the argument that contemporary society produces such a density of symbols and meanings that they have become detached from their original locations and take on a life of their own, Baudrillard goes on to argue that an important consequence of this is a quality of reversibility. Thus, one can collect, by moving forwards and backwards across lifestyles that were previously temporally located, symbols and meanings from which to create an identity. Identity is no longer contingent on the organizing principle of the lifecourse. Identities may be adopted and discarded over time, not as a consequence of any sense of progression or development, but at the caprice of the wearer. One can, at least in theory, hit the fast-forward and rewind buttons of life in order to cast the ageing process into oblivion.

Writers such as Featherstone and Hepworth (1989) have made considerable use of this and similar analyses to gain an understanding of postmodern ageing. They note that postmodern change has led to a 'blurring of what appeared previously to be relatively clearly marked stages and the experiences and characteristic behaviour which were associated with those stages' (Featherstone and Hepworth 1989: 144). These trends include a focus on the fluidity of social images and expectations with respect to an ageing identity. Key to these new imaginal possibilities would be the relationship between body and identity and, most notably, a rejection of deterministic narratives in favour of the elder as a consumer of more youthful lifestyle choices. However, reversibility also condemns human development, as an anthropologist, Lee (1998), points out, to a hinterland of 'betwixt and between periods' typical of rites of passage in traditional societies, and in which the normal rules of social organization are suspended. These periods of indeterminate identity have been translated, by Baudrillard, into a continuous state of affairs. Transition, in other words, is a trip from which Baudrillard fails to come down. A lifecourse is presented which can offer no sense of purpose or direction other than as a continuing round of interchangeability that only death can stop (Baudrillard 1993).

Faced with such possibilities, Bauman (1995: 81) suggests that the questions asked of identity development also change. 'If the modern "problem of identity" was how to construct an identity and keep it solid and stable', he claims, 'the postmodern "problem of identity" is primarily how to avoid fixation and keep the options open. In the case of identity as in other cases, the catchword for modernity was "creation"; the catchword of postmodernity is "recycling".' Reading Bauman, it appears that rather than trying to hold something of the lifecourse solid and continuous, strategies for identity consist of a persistent desire to escape that responsibility. Life is best kept fragmentary and episodic, because a life lived as a succession of episodes is freed from the worry about consequences.

Episodic encounters are enacted 'as if they had no past history and no future; whatever there is to the encounter, tends to be begotten and exhausted in the span of the encounter itself' (Bauman 1995: 49). The personal lifecourse is played, according to this perspective, with the intention of inconsequentiality, so that the past cannot come to haunt the players and life is experienced in a continuous present. Under these conditions, Bauman argues that previous life strategies no longer hold. There is little point in building for the future if there is no guarantee that what is valued today will be seen the same way tomorrow. Rather, people attempt to protect themselves through the creation of an as-if world, likened to the tourist who 'everywhere he goes he is in, but nowhere of the place', and cannot be touched by what goes on there. In this world, ageing becomes an experience of observing the exotic and grotesque while 'keeping hope alive by the expedient of indefinite postponement' (Bauman 1995: 49).

The conception of identity emerging from consumerism and its corollaries in episodic and reversible self-presentation has had particular implications for the lifecourse. Kumar (1995) has suggested, for example, that self and personal identity have now to be conceived as spatial rather than historical entities, with the consequence that there is now no expectation of continuous lifelong development, and no story of personal growth over time. If personal biography becomes a matter of discontinuous experiences and identities, there is no need for the narrative of a developing personality. There are stories of the self in this model, but they function to lend plausablility to whichever identity is currently being performed. Their purpose is short-term, and is supplied, in Giddens's (1991) phrase, simply to 'keep a particular narrative going'. This process applies as much to the future as it does to the past, as one's plans, as well as one's past story, contribute to the convincingness of the current episode. To keep a current narrative going over time denies the effects of time itself. The story is made up and contingent upon an experience of a continuous present tense. It must contain processes that allow the weathering of current transitions, riding them out, surfing their waves; and, in this, continuity over time has been replaced by the feeling of continuousness. In such ways, it is suggested, consumer culture supplies the props and the environment, allowing the construction of an eternal present with no centre, origin or destination.

A quite novel perspective on the lifecourse, and thus adult identity, appears to emerge from this analysis. For, rather than there being the maintenance of a continuous and historically embedded core to the personality, it is suggested that the concerns traditionally associated with an ageing identity can be avoided. Further, this is no longer an argument over the eclipsing of ageing and its discontent through a consumer culture preoccupied with youth. It is suggested instead that ageing can effectively be abolished. This is achieved through entry into a series of episodes, buoyed up by the consumption of appropriate props, thus allowing the deployment of a variety of identities.

HITTING THE BUFFERS

It would seem that a fundamental shift is being suggested in the debate on ageing and identity. It takes the form of a move away from an examination of threats to the self occasioned by changes in age status. Instead, ageing increasingly becomes a matter of consumer choice and contingent identities, which might be repeatedly recycled and thereby ensure continued social inclusion. This restatement of the problem would also question the continued relevance of signs of ageing in positioning older people in society, as signs may no longer signify anything greater than what social actors want them to. To search for genuineness in age-related identities might become meaningless if each identity becomes as synthetic as its neighbour.

Even the body, which Butler (1987) suggested was an undeniable sign of age, thus giving permission to ageist attitudes, is malleable under postmodern conditions. Falk (1995), for example, proposes that the body now takes on the role of a surface which can be 'intentionally elaborated', raw material that can be worked on. In later life, Featherstone and Wernick (1995: 3) suggest, it is now possible to 'recode the body itself' as biomedical and information technology make available 'The capacity to alter not just the meaning, but the very material infrastructure of the body. Bodies can be reshaped, remade, fused with machines, empowered through technological devices and extensions.'

A focus on a new and flexible interpretation of the body becomes key to understanding both images of ageing and identity management. It promises an escape from deterministic and age-related limits similar to the way that consumerism allows the mature adult to buy his or her way out of age-stereotyping and, on first reading, both factors appear to

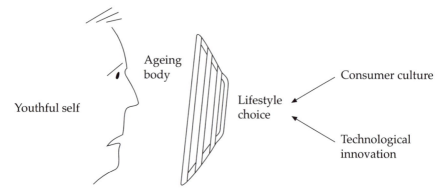

Figure 3.1   The 'mask of ageing'.

suggest an increase in the possibilities for identity choice in later life. It is also here, however, that the project of maintaining multiple options for identity hits the buffers of ageing as a physical process. For even though the postmodern 'self' is characterized as being capable of infinite expression, the ageing body needs to be progressively managed if this possibility is not to be lost. Old age increases this contradiction to a point at which participation in consumer lifestyles is significantly compromised. As ageing gathers pace, it is increasingly difficult to 'recycle' the body and it becomes a cage, which both entraps and denies access to that world of choice.

In terms of positioning the question of maturity, this line of reasoning suggests that the core problem lies between the maintenance of an ageing identity and an individual's own body. Featherstone and Hepworth (1990: 255) have suggested that one way of understanding this process requires the perception of bodily ageing as a mask 'which cannot be removed: any connection they may have with the individual's personal sense of identity is the result of the ways other people react to changes in facial appearance and the social categories they imply.' Thus, social actors discover discontinuity between the mask of ageing, as found in an increasingly unattractive and unresponsive body, and their actual desires and sense of self (see Figure 3.1).

Hepworth (1991: 93) positions this contradiction in terms of inner youthfulness and bodily age: 'At the heart of the difficulty of explaining what it's like to be old lies the awareness of an experiential difference between the physical processes of ageing, as reflected in outward appearance, and the inner or subjective "real self" which paradoxically remains young.' This relationship has been described by Turner (1995) as a betrayal of the youthfulness of an 'inner body', and, in order to re-establish a link with consumerism and the choice of identity that it implies, something has to be done about the ageing body as that thing that 'conceals the enduring and more youthful self' (Featherstone and Hepworth 1990). The mask motif and the problem of ageing, then, are couched in terms of an antagonism between the ageing body and a youthful 'inner' self. The body, while it is malleable, can still provide access to a variety of consumer identities. However, as Biggs (1997c) notes, it leads to an end-game in which older people are at war with themselves, an internalized battle between the psyche and the body in which the social aspects of an ageing identity have been lost. Ageing has become a nightmare stalking the postmodern consumer's utopia, and reverses its libertarian possibilities. It produces a contradiction between the fixedness of the body and the fluidity of social images. It tells the tourist that it is time to go home and the Peter and Petra Pans that there may be an unpalatable end to their story.

SUMMARY AND IMPLICATIONS

A considerable tension is emerging here between the mature identity imagined by psychodynamic thinking and ideas about consumer identities and the ageing self. While moves towards understanding the importance of relationships, the here and now and multiple identity have moved psychotherapy on to similar ground to postmodern thinking, its model is still closely identified with the notion of a core self that needs nurturing and maintenance across a variety of unstable settings. It also appears that a relaxation of preoccupations with childhood in psychotherapy has happened simultaneously to the proposal of a youthful self trapped within an ageing body. This constitutes a surprising reversal of the tasks of mature identity, now seen through the lens of postmodern consumer culture. On the one hand it is assumed that an authentic adult identity can be understood by concentrating on immediate experience; on the other, that the immediate experience of ageing is an impediment to the emergence of a genuine and youthful identity. Instead of elders escaping the contradictions of early experience, youthful identity has re-emerged as a wistfully desired and immanently threatened state.

Along the way, a lot of established markers have been jettisoned. These include the eschewal of longitudinal experience as a basis for identity. Adult identity has been construed as a series of fragmented episodes, which by their very disconnectedness protect the player from unwelcome consequences. The personal past now functions as a bin full of decontextualized source material, from which the needs for current identities can be met. The past has become a metaphor for the present, which itself draws on rather than reflects a remembrance of a personal history. Neither does it seem necessary to worry about keeping the self intact.

Multiple identities provide an ultimate defence against the assaults of contemporary ageing, as they allow the individual to move on, and keep moving on if difficulties are faced. This appears to be a complex world of successive identities, each as valid as its predecessor. It is one in which concern for coherence and an emphasis on consolidation evaporate, because discontinuities between age and identities no longer matter.

The postmodern is not a perspective that makes clear distinctions between personal fantasy, intersubjective constructions and historical and emotional memory. At a personal level, it becomes increasingly difficult to distinguish between wants and needs. It appears unnecessary to distinguish the authentic from the inauthentic. It throws into contention a need for rooted coherence and is marked by superficial relations with others. Authenticity is, however, important from a psychodynamic perspective, both for a durable and convincing sense of self, and as a criterion for experience to be handed on to others who might learn lessons from it. If neither of these criteria applies, reflection on the significance of ageing and the role of intergenerational communication becomes meaningless. The possibility of learning from history and of intergenerational solidarity is diminished.

Two versions of an ageing identity emerge from this debate. A psychodynamic view might hold that, having knocked away the established props for an embedded identity, the mature imagination requires internal coherence in order to negotiate an increasingly uncertain world. The postmodern perspective embraces social fragmentation as a source of newly made and unmade identities. Consumer culture can furnish lifestyles and adaptations to the ageing body to keep this chimeric process alive. However, it has to reinvent a distinction between the hidden and the apparent in order to explain ageing away as the disguising of a youthful inner self. Whereas the psychodynamic, and most notably Jungian, model sees the inner life as the manifestation of mature adulthood, the postmodern adult psyche is really an indeterminately young and possibly ageless person trying to get out. In answer to the question of how age should be thought of, postmodernity at first denies its relevance, then sees it as a threat to unlimited hedonism. The subjectivity of mature adulthood is conceived of as youthful potential trapped in an ageing container, and it is therefore questionable whether experience intrinsic to maturity is at all considered.

4

Masque and ageing

HIDDEN AND SURFACE

Consideration of the relationship between ageing and identity has produced two antagonistic and possibly incompatible demands. On the one
hand, a need emerges to protect the mature imagination from hostile and
fragmenting conceptions of the lifecourse. On the other, a celebration of
surface, consumerism and reversibility invites the possibility of eliminating many of the consequences of ageing altogether. The traditional psychoanalytic solution to problems of identity has been to quell, or attempt to
quell, internal monsters through re-experiencing events that gave them
birth. The object has been to reconcile base emotions to the civilizing force
of social cohesion. This task defines the nature and purpose of the adult
imagination. Ego psychology extended this argument by focusing on the
shaping of consciousness through successive tasks of self-definition. The
outcome of this approach was further to embed the process of ageing
into a fixed set of social conditions. Analytical psychology set a separate
path, centred on increasing inner coherence, thereby effecting a transition
from the priorities of younger adulthood to those of the second half of
life and discovering new existential goals in maturity.

The debate over modernity and postmodern conditions has drawn attention to three elements that have been underplayed in this psychodynamic
sketch of the adult lifecourse. The first of these is that ageing takes place
in a potentially hostile environment which spans a continuum. At one
end, emphasis on production relegates adults who are not in work and
older people in particular to a marginal position in society, while at the
other a focus on the role of consumption in maintaining identities places
adults in an antagonistic position towards their ageing bodies. Under
these circumstances, technologies of self such as the psychotherapies can
no longer sustain a resort solely to conformity or its destructive status,

once these contradictions in the relationship between self-development and the social constructions of adulthood have been identified. Second, contemporary society is, in its very composition, subject to radical and continuous change. This has meant that the mature imagination requires techniques that maintain some form of stable selfhood through a paradoxical adoption of the processes of continual becoming. Theories that have been used to describe the adult lifecourse can now themselves be seen as attempts to fix identity or embrace diversity in this dizzying and fragmenting environment. Any settlement is made contingent on the ability of identity to stay afloat in this uncertain world. Third, resolutions to the 'problem of ageing' that emerge through postmodernity, while initially celebrating a diversity of surface identities, episodes and lifestyles, have had to reinvent the division between the hidden and the surface in adult psychology to engage with the questions that ageing presents. Life cannot simply be seen as consisting of surfaces and impressions 'all the way down'. There is an inner self which stubbornly re-emerges, either as younger or as more developed than appearances would suggest, and whose relationship to the consumption of 'identity statements' is rendered problematic by age.

This reinvention of the hidden, required by the particular challenges of later life, has resulted in psychodynamic and postmodern perspectives becoming increasingly interdependent if contemporary ageing is to be understood. Without the grounding influence of psychodynamic thinking, postmodern theorizing results in trajectory without teleology. It has movement without direction and makes a virtue out of disconnection. Age, however, connects identity with finitude. The limited span of life, a progressive need to manage the body and a culture hostile to the mature imagination raise existential questions that render revelling in consumption shallow and without purpose. Without recognition of the looseness of contents and the multiple options that exist under postmodern conditions, psychodynamic thinking succumbs to the dangers of ossification and a serious misreading of the issues facing mature integrity.

CONTINUITY AND COHESION

These new conditions challenge the very language used to articulate the ageing process. An example can be seen in the notion of development itself. Development is closely linked to ideas of progress across the lifecourse, an idea that has now become contested territory. Development suggests linear movement over time, a progression based on increasing chronological age, from which identity obtains some form of continuity. However, a change of emphasis to the consumption of a multiplicity of episodes, experienced as taking place in a continuous present, leaves little space for the apprehension of this type of continuity. Rather, if there is a debate beyond shopping until dropping, a shift in attention is suggested towards the nature and value of cohesion; whether, in other words, the constructed identity holds together at any one point in time. Continuity suggests form through the apprehension of consistent patterning across the lifecourse, and its opposite, discontinuity, registers changes in direction but does not displace an underlying acceptance of temporal progression. Cohesion, on the other hand, privileges the association of qualities, unpeeled and subject to recombination. These are simultaneously available within time frames that fail to register deep-seated yet slow-moving mutability.

One of the results of these conceptual changes in emphasis, then, has been that coherence of identity is increasingly seen as a matter of cohesion rather than continuity. Traditional psychoanalysis has drawn heavily on progression and repetition over time and thus the framework of continuity, while attention to the here and now brings with it a concern that aspects of the self are sufficiently flexible but still make sense as a story about the self. Personal coherence becomes an issue of whether the 'glue' that holds personality together has become too rigid or too flexible, rather than whether the timetable makes sense.

Questions raised by these new conditions have considerable importance for our understanding of age and the challenges it presents. Is it important, for example, to achieve coherence through continuity, and should continuity be rooted in a 'real' past or simply serve to fuel a particular narrative of a supposed past? Can a sense of personal becoming be maintained in inhospitable social circumstances, and if so how are the protective spaces that allow this to happen to be maintained? These spaces would be both psychological in nature, maintained by strategies for identity management, and related to material spaces, consisting of buildings, clothing, lifestyles, available in the external world. Further, within these questions lies the problem of whether, and how, a more genuine, self-identified focus for consciousness is hidden beyond appearances and the multiplicity inherent in consumer culture.

APPEARANCE AND AUTHENTICITY

While the models of adult identity identified above differ in the priority given to surface or depth, with postmodern models of identity privileging the former and psychodynamic models the latter, a tension between appearance and authenticity is carried by both. In Featherstone and Hepworth's (1991, 1995) proposal for a 'mask of ageing', it is the ageing body that masks the inner and youthful self. This model suggests that continuity is maintained by a youthful or timeless identity, while discontinuity is experienced through the 'progressive betrayals of the body' that have been associated with age. In the case of the mask of ageing, a solution appears in the use of various props and technological advances. These would include the use of virtual reality, communication on an anonymized (at least in terms of appearance) Internet, the modification of the body itself through prosthesis and cyborgic machine–body combinations (Haraway 1991). The ageing body itself becomes masked through a theoretical, and in some cases practical, return to the delights of a particular form of techno-biological consumerism. By contrast, psychological models based on the idea that ageing takes the form of progressively individuated maturation (Tornstam 1994, 1996; Biggs 1993a, 1997c) tend to place the ageing self behind a mask rooted in social conformity. Continuity is more easily held by the body as the physical centre of personal experience, while the self is marked by transcendent change. In these approaches, inspired in part by analytic psychology, it is the self that experiences the discontinuity of the first and second halves of life and expands as a result of new challenges and new psychological contents becoming available to consciousness. In Jung's own thinking, however, the role of the social mask, or persona, was significantly underdeveloped, the principle task of therapy being to enhance the mature and active imagination. The persona was assumed to fall away with age. It was associated not with body at all, but with the conceit of social position. Neither tradition has developed a considered analysis of the strategies that mature adults might adopt to negotiate a meaningful place in their social worlds. Such strategies would need to take both surface appearances and hidden aspects of identity into account.

The absence of a developed understanding of the processes underpinning the strategic and tactical negotiation of an ageing identity is, then, not simply the result of ageist assumptions of later life as a time of passivity and rigidity. These are the views that one becomes stuck in one's ways, incapable of creative energy, dependent on the second-hand roles ascribed to age by younger generations or the workings of capital. Important as they are, these forces coexist with conceptual understandings of age that have paid little attention to the creation and maintenance of a mature identity. Instead, age has been cast into a dynamic of fixity and change that can now be seen as a possibly false dichotomy. Within this schema, the fixedness of social conformity, an unresponsive body and an old dog bemused by new tricks are set against the opportunities and uncertainties of personal expansion and mix 'n' match consumer display. Fixedness and change are seen as opposites or alternative positions that can be adopted in response to adult ageing. However, it might be the case that the negotiations and accommodations tacit in the maintenance of mature adulthood require an amalgam of both fixity and change. There might, then, be aspects of the mature imagination that lend stability, through continuity and cohesion, as well as an ability to adapt flexibly and play creatively with personal identity. Under contemporary conditions, an adaptive and mature self might contain an interplay of depth and surface, hidden and apparent, fixed positions and flexible change in order to negotiate social processes of ageing. Indeed, an interplay of depth, surface and degrees of coherence allows different, yet complementary, processes of self-definition to take place simultaneously. A more complex and ultimately more satisfying model of maturity, which acts to preserve and protect continuity of self development while at the same time adapting to the opportunities and demands of multiple and episodic environments, can emerge.

AN EXPERIENTIAL SPLIT

There are a number of reports in the literature that indicate an experiential split between appearance and a sense of selfhood in later life. And while these often refer to physical change, this is by no means the only, or most profound, manifestation of this disjuncture. An examination of the positions explored by authors in this area might illuminate ways in which tensions between hidden and surface, fixity and change, are worked out in maturity.

Perhaps the best known reference to this phenomenon has been made by Simone de Beauvoir (1970). She indicates that the ageing self as other has its roots not in the experience of age itself, but in younger adults' inability to imagine continuity between their current selves and themselves in later life. 'The characteristic mark of the adult's attitude toward the old is its duplicity', she states (de Beauvoir 1970: 245), meaning that while younger adults, most notably the older adult's own children, officially respect age-seniority, they will also seek to undermine and ultimately supplant their parents. The lineage of this argument is oedipal and, according to de Beauvoir, leads to a climate of manipulation and subtle undermining of the mature adult's position. This sense that later life is alien to younger adults and may present a barrier, manifested by others, to their own achievement contributes to the experience of personal ageing as divided: 'Can I have become a different being while I still remain myself?' (de Beauvoir 1970: 315). De Beauvoir considered the view that a solution based on 'feeling young inside' was an outsider's misunderstanding of this dilemma. Rather, it is the 'person I am for the outsider' who is considered old, to which 'no challenge is permissible'. This argument is continued by discussion of a mistaken correspondence between ageing and disease and the view that 'Modern society, far from providing the aged man with an appeal against his biological fate, tosses him into an outdated past, and it does so while he is still living' (de Beauvoir 1970: 423).

De Beauvoir's solution to the challenges of ageing is to maintain existential projects, which are both a continuation of interests and causes throughout life and an adaptation to new social circumstances. Her publication of *La Viellesse* at age 62 can be seen as an example of the combination of continuing concerns and new conditions. She continues: 'There is only one solution if old age is not to be an absurd parody of our former life, and that is to go on pursuing ends that give our experience meaning', by which is meant 'devotion to individuals, to groups or to causes, social, political intellectual or creative work' (de Beauvoir 1970: 601). So, according to de Beauvoir, the challenges of intergenerational rivalry, which lead to the dominant perspectives of ageing as disease and outmoded experience, result in an antagonistic relationship between personal projects and socially constructed age. She exhorts the continuing pursuit of projects which are appropriate to later life, and thus not 'an absurd parody', and at the same time maintain relatedness to wider social issues.

The positive value of political commitment in later life has been examined by Andrews (1991). She relates long-term activism to optimism and the recognition of a Freiresque (Freire 1972) oppressor within, which one has to come to terms with and grow beyond. An encounter with internalized stereotypes of others, and latterly oneself, is noted as an important transformative step in consciousness. Thus, 'Psychological development and the commitment to work for social change are not antithetical.' It is argued that, in the lives of the 15 political activists studied, 'These two processes have been one and the same' (Andrews 1991: 206). Disjuncture between social appearance and an internal apprehension of mature identity can also be found in the work of Thompson (1992). His study of subjective ageing, 'I don't feel old', indicates that a rejection of 'old' does not necessarily imply a rejection of the experience of ageing. Rather, it is an act of 'defiance of a spoiled identity' which 'demands an exceptional ability to respond imaginatively to change' (Thompson 1992: 27). It is, in other words, the stereotype, rather than the experience, that is contested. People use the label 'old' to describe negative experiences associated with ageing, rather than ageing itself. He notes that post-retirement activities are remarkably diverse. Further, for intimate adult relations, 'later life is a time when these relationships need to be continually rebuilt. In this it is more like youth than the middle years of life' (Thompson 1992: 35).

The view that emerges from these observations is that an ageing identity requires a relatedness and flexibility which is sufficiently resilient to repulse ageist attack. There is an intimation that the mature imagination works at more than one level in the puzzle of remaining oneself, while simultaneously becoming different. The relationship between personal expression and social emancipation is a theme which underwrites much of the discussion of masque and social space in this book. Personal strategies by which this is achieved, however, have only been lightly drawn and require a further empirical and conceptual exploration for their elaboration.

SOCIAL RELATIONS AND MATURE IDENTITY

Social relationships in later life have been reviewed by Phillipson (1997), who notes a research focus on three main areas: family life, marital relationships and friendship patterns. It is concluded that relationships are becoming increasingly diverse in form and that supportive peer relationships are of great importance to a sense of well-being. Family commitments are, as observed by Finch (1995), subject to negotiation and depend on the quality of a particular relationship to a larger degree than previously thought. Coleman (1996), in an extensive review of identity management in later life, comments on the power of transformation which the perceiving self is able to wield in the interpretation of and adaptation to adversity. He concludes that there is a growing research consensus that 'personality traits tend to be stable with age, whereas key aspects of the self, such as goals, values, coping styles and control beliefs are more amenable to change' (Coleman 1996: 97). A managed identity can achieve continuity through role changes, stigma and threats to physical integrity, which Atchley (1989, 1991) identifies with 'a more tested and stable set of processes for self management and more robust self concepts'. Coleman also draws attention to the importance of 'domain specific self-concepts' (Lachman 1986; Markus and Nurius 1986), which allow responding to vary between contexts and categories. He suggests that these characteristics allow for defence against the negative attitudes of others and that, 'Although the changes associated with age are perceived almost uniformly negatively, most older people maintain high levels of wellbeing, preventing their fears from being recognised by coping successfully with the threats that come their way' (Coleman 1996: 107).

Successful ageing is, in other words, marked by heterogeneity, which is often the result of an interplay between processes of selection, compensation and optimization (Baltes and Carstensen 1996). This position is reflected in Kastenbaum's (1993) observation that creativity in maturity requires achievement of a balance between the desire to encompass a wide variety of expression and the control of expression within a coherent structure, and in Cohler's (1993) observation that maintaining a coherent narrative is itself a strategy for the management of meaning and sustaining morale. Feinstein (1997) suggests that personal myths, or narratives, are self-consciously modified as they become self-limiting with age and require adaptive transformation. To these can be added Chinen's (1989) reports from psychotherapy that capacities develop with increasing maturity, from a period of 'youthful cleverness' marked by linear direction and self-confidence, through a pragmatic problem-solving phase, to more holistic and metaphysical preoccupations.

In this context it is interesting to note Gubrium's (1993) research, and, in particular, observations on the manner in which experience is given voice. Throughout, older adults emerge as careful listeners (Gubrium and Wallace 1990). Gubrium suggests that an 'it depends' quality to responding does not indicate an absence of decision-making, but rather deliberation over a number of possible alternatives. It 'Indicates that respondents precede their answers with questions of their own about experiential contingencies and that answers to these questions condition what is eventually conveyed as responses to inquiries. The "it depends" quality of answers implies that the respondent can voice diverse senses of the personal experiences being studied, varying by narrative context' (Gubrium 1993: 48). This conditional quality of mature discourse is, it is contended, often missed by directive research agendas which overlook its public or social quality. It is, in other words, a sign of 'savvy people' whose responding in groups to a helping professional varies considerably, depending on the relevance of their expertise to the topic under discussion, and could become anti-professional, or attentive to expert opinion, depending on context. These conclusions are similar to Biggs's (1993a) critical reappraisal of groupwork, undertaken to examine older adults' communication styles, which may by turns reflect resistance, intolerance or a sharing of younger adults' agendas.

A view emerges, from these reports, of maturity as a time in which experienced social actors draw on a variety of techniques and stratagems in order to maintain a developing identity. Indeed, as physical sources of status wane, it makes some evolutionary sense that other, more sophisticated, methods come to hand to retain some form of personal control. By the time mature adulthood is reached, the psyche has at its disposal the pragmatism of multiple responding, plus an increasing sense of personal coherence which retains a sense of both masquerade and the profound. It may thus be able to deploy identity very much in the way of a performance.

COMING TO THE MASQUERADE

The use of a metaphor of masquerade to examine ageing and experience can be seen in the work of the poet W. B. Yeats (Ellman 1949; Webster 1973). Yeats devised his own cosmology, in which individual development consisted of attributes dramatized as their opposites, thus concealing a more intimate self. For Yeats, the mask was an ambivalent construct, which allowed for the expression of personal presence and personality that the wearer wished for, yet was a creation of artifice. Of particular interest is Yeats's attribution of his continued creativity in old age to the presence of the mask and to an increased sense of personal wholeness (Pruitt 1982). However, in this literary source, the mask is often used rhetorically and was not clearly elaborated as a social strategy. Drama-turgical analogies have been used by Goffman (1960, 1967) to examine the presentation of self. Some authors (Tseelon 1992, 1995; Smart 1993) have drawn on Goffman's preoccupation with impression management as a manipulation of social surfaces to elaborate postmodern forms of identity. However, for present purposes, Goffman's work fails to engage, with the possible exception of his examination of stigma (1963), with the interplay of hiddenness, depth and social conformity. It is, as a number of authors (Gergen 1991; Tseelon 1992; Biggs 1997c) have observed, as if Goffman's actors have no interior or exterior, they simply keep supportive interchanges going.

More recent employment of a masking motif can be found in the work of both exponents and critics of postmodernism. Jameson (1984: 65), for example, identifies the postmodern condition with the eclipse of parody by pastiche. 'Pastiche is, like parody, the intimation of a peculiar mask, speech in a dead language: but it is a neutral practice of such mimicry, without any of parody's ulterior motives . . . Pastiche is thus blank parody.' Style eclipses substance, surface, depth, and with a waning of affect, there is no space for the outward dramatization of inner feeling. The postmodern use of mask, it is argued, fails to look any deeper than the masquerade itself. This view finds some confirmation in Baudrillard's (in Sandywell 1995) outline of successive and loosely historical phases in how representation, of which the relationship between masquerade and social reality is an example, has been perceived. These begin by describ-ing representations as reflections of a pre-given and basic reality. Then, with increased abstraction, masks emerge which pervert reality and dis-guise some underlying truth. Following this phase, representations are said to mask the absence of any coherent reality, and finally an environ-ment in which distinctions between the real and the unreal themselves become meaningless. This description reflects the now familiar post-modern argument that appearances no longer signify anything other than their own surface meanings. However, it has been given a novel and unexpected twist by Bauman (1997), who argues that in the absence of determining narratives, which in this case would include those pertaining to a defined trajectory for middle and old age, individuals are thrown back upon their own resources. They are required to take responsibility for their own actions and fashion their own identities precisely because grand narratives and defined representations are no longer reliably avail-able. According to Bauman, masquerade can, under these conditions, become another means of avoiding personal responsibility. Masks might simply reflect short-term episodes of identity which embody an art of forgetting and interchangeability rather than remembrance and continuity.

The most sustained critical employment of the masquerade motif can be found in feminist discourses on gender. Here, the contradictions of feminized identities have given rise, it is argued, to masking as contested territory, including both conformity and resistance to gender stereotyping. The relationship between masquerade and femininity has been noted by a number of authors (Nava 1992; Tseelon 1995; Lury 1996), with an emphasis on an ability to engage in and subvert dominant identity statements through performance and play. 'Artificiality', states Tseelon (1995: 34), 'is not threatening in itself. It is a means to an end.' The debate is framed, she notes, in terms of whether 'decorativeness, fashions, beauty procedures' are external to the self or indicative of an inauthenticity of character. Tseelon criticizes the approach of the psychoanalyst Jean Riviere (1929), who associated feminine masquerade with a hidden and unconscious masculinity in women, but did not fully reject masking as a civilizing process. This is unsurprising, as it was Riviere who suggested the title *Civilization and Its Discontents* to Freud for his own related work. Tseelon (1995: 38) continues that, with the growth of urban society, 'Masks became a device for creating a private sphere, even in public. Not surprisingly this coincided with the emergence of the public masquerade which combined desire for public interaction with keeping private boundaries intact.' However, she points out that while masquerade appears to challenge fixed, and in this case patriarchal, definitions of identity, it remains dependent on that dominant frame of reference. A masque is therefore double-edged. It simultaneously disguises and draws attention to what it tries to hide, just as the process of disguise itself has elements of spectacle. The suggestion of hidden otherness is a continuing theme in work of this genre and extends to the artwork of Cindy Sherman, who photographs herself in a variety of roles and attitudes in order to unveil what Mulvey (1991) has described as the use of the female body as a metaphor of division between 'surface allure and concealed decay'. Butler (1996) proposes that gender is by its nature performative, then extends this logic to suggest that performance is 'radically free' insofar as the 'materiality of the body is vacated or ignored'. She promotes 'transgressive performances' such as drag to destabilize traditional gender categories. According to Butler, one is defined as much by what one is not as by the position that is explicitly inhabited.

In many cases the deployment of masquerade has been mediated by age. Thus, Matthews (1979) observed that older women actively managed the information they gave to younger people, trying simultaneously to maintain a positive view of themselves and the adoption of an age-free identity. Older women, she argued, had one identity for other people and one for themselves. A presentation of self dependent on the age of the other has also been reported by Coupland *et al.* (1991). They note that 'vividly contrasting age identities' were created by an older woman, with a more assertive, lively and elaborated presentation of self among peers than that shaped between her and a younger woman. Viewed in this light, strategies of painful self-disclosure and spontaneous telling of age, observed by Giles and Coupland (1991) in daycare settings, may function to maintain intergenerational distance. They describe interaction at a sufficiently superficial level to ensure the smooth running of communication, and insulate both parties from the threat of more intrusive and sustained contact. They are, in other words, a mask.

Latimer (1997) has studied the elaborate performances that professionals and patients adopt in hospital settings and concludes that conforming identities may simply denote the most effective strategy available to older patients in achieving desired outcomes, rather than being an expression of more genuine and deep seated desires. In other, non-service settings, Healey (1994) has indicated that a common strategy among older women is to try to 'pass' as being from a younger age-group. She notes the costs of such a strategy of pretence: 'in passing you are saying that who you are at sixty, seventy, eighty, is not ok. You are ok only to the degree that you are like someone else' (Healey 1994: 82). It follows that it is difficult to address both the process of ageing, at least in public, and the creation of a more genuine ageing identity. This view is supported by Ingrisch (1995), who suggests a conformity to social expectations coexisting with suppressed wishes and longings in her interviews with 30 women in old age. Identity, for these women, was marked by a tension between conformity and resistance to perceived social expectation.

Woodward (1991) specifically discusses the role of masquerade in later life. For her, masquerade is a form of self-representation that 'has to do with concealing something and presenting the very conditions of that concealment'. Thus, 'masquerade entails several strategies, among them: the addition of desired body-parts (teeth, hair); the removal or covering up of unwanted parts of the body (growths, gray hair, "age-spots"); the lifting of the face and other body parts in an effort to deny the weight of gravity; the moulding of the body's shape (exercise, clothing)' (Woodward 1991: 148).

In the deployment of the masque, youth becomes a normative state to which the body has to be restored. Age becomes a process of dispossession and the cover-up, an exercise teetering on the brink of the grotesque. Through this intrinsic ambiguity, masquerade again becomes a process of submission to dominant social codes and resistance to them. Woodward's observation that masquerade in later life involves concealment and pretence, and is at the same time an expression of the ageing condition, emphasizes the reflexivity of masking in this context. It is a thing that is played with, which while obscuring signs of ageing is also drawing attention to the fact that a deceit is taking place. In other words, the mask is not the same as the person underneath and 'tells a certain truth of its own'. Woodward (1991: 148) also links masking and external attacks on the self: 'In a culture which so devalues age, masquerade with respect to the ageing body is first and foremost a denial of age, an effort to erase or efface age and to put on youth.'

However, it is often unclear from these observations whether one is engaging primarily in a discourse on youth rather than the subjectivity of old age. The physicality of feminine masquerade, centred on the visual and the body, leads masking to be understood first and foremost as a concrete phenomenon which is prioritized over other forms of presentation. Resistance appears cloaked in the melancholic and the grotesque, a theatre of old bodies playing at youth; whereas for others youth can be put on like a summer dress. We do not, however, change bodies as Baudrillard and Butler would somewhat breezily have us believe. A somewhat enigmatic affirmation that this process simultaneously reveals and disguises requires further elaboration. It appears unclear whether this simultaneity is a failure of the 'youthful' project, a subtle play or parody on the ambiguity of a mature imagination or a source of Foucauldian resistance to an established order. Masquerade alone can be seen as an attempt to manipulate this intersubjectivity and achieve a balance between the personally real and the disguise.

THE USES OF PERSONA

The persona is an essentially social phenomenon which encompasses the roles we play and the compromises we make for the sake of 'fitting in'. It expresses accommodations the psyche makes to social requirements, the adoption of social conventions in order to be taken seriously by other participants in social discourse, to be given a legitimized voice. The metaphor arises from the use of masks in classical theatre, which disguised the actor, described a character and amplified the voice. In analytical psychology, it describes a way in which identity is presented in acceptable ways to others. From this perspective, the work of Goffman and other symbolic interactionists would be seen as elaborations of the persona. Neither is the mask as persona primarily physical, although habitual and repetitive performance may shape the contours of the face and body. The persona is a device through which an active self looks out at and negotiates with the world, to protect the self and to deceive others.

It has already been mentioned that Jung was not overly concerned with the persona, perceiving it as a diversion from a true understanding of the individual self. As a result, he left it conceptually underdeveloped. 'The persona is a complicated system of relations between individual consciousness and society, fittingly enough, a kind of mask, designed on the one hand to make a definite impression upon others and on the other to conceal the true nature of the individual' (Jung 1967b: 303). He also believed that, 'Fundamentally, the persona is nothing real, it is a compromise between individual and society as to what man should appear to be' (Jung 1967b: 158).

Contemporary descriptions of persona have concentrated on a number of aspects of its function. First, the persona is now seen to hold positive qualities that facilitate social interaction. It acts as a bridge between the social and the personal. Frieda Fordham (1956: 49) notes, for example, that 'It simplifies our contacts by indicating what we may expect from other people and on the whole makes them pleasanter, as good clothes improve ugly bodies.' As Samuels *et al.* (1986: 107) say, 'There is an inevitability and ubiquity to persona . . . involving all the compromises appropriate to living in a community.' According to this view, the persona is a necessary part of social life, making life more predictable, protecting the self and others from less acceptable or 'ugly' parts of people's personalities that might inhibit day-to-day social exchange. The social world is taken as a given in such an interpretation. For while these authors, especially Samuels (1993), welcome the extension of analytical psychology to broader social concerns, little consideration is given to the construction of social space, why some characteristics of individuals are accepted and others not, except through the mechanism of the individual repression of inconvenient beliefs and attitudes. The persona may fulfil the important function of connecting inner and outer worlds, of grounding personal fantasies in social reality, but it extracts the price of social conformity.

A second perspective continues the theme of social accommodation as problematic. This line of thought expands upon Jung's original observation that the persona restricts self-development and thus genuine communication. Particular attention has been paid to over-identification with the persona, such that social actors mistake the mask for genuine personal identity. Samuels (1984, 1993) describes adopting a rigid persona as being undertaken at significant cost to personal development, most notably through an inability to own aspects of the personality that might conflict with the social mask, and the projection of unacceptable parts of the self on to others. Further, over-identification with the mask eclipses depth and awareness of internal influences on behaviour. 'The ego, when it is identified with the persona is capable only of external orientation. It is blind to internal events and hence unable to respond to them . . . It follows that it is possible to remain unconscious of one's persona' (Samuels *et al.* 1986: 93). These conditions can lead either to a feeling that social interaction 'has merely the value of an amusing playground' (Jung 1967b: 199) in which no commitments are binding and nothing touches the self, or to a position in which the mask becomes increasingly mistaken for the whole of personal identity. Thus, if social actors express themselves primarily through social masking, the mask can become fixed, welded to consciousness so completely that one becomes unaware of other potential avenues for self-expression, and even that one is wearing a mask at all. In other words, one exists in a world of surfaces.

Elsewhere (Biggs 1997c) it has been argued that thinking of the mask as a bridge and as a betrayal of self-expression has underplayed a third key function of persona performances. The social mask does not simply disguise, it also protects the wearer from assaults to personal identity arising from inhospitable social circumstances. Professional helpers, for example, who have to perform socially necessary yet personally challenging tasks as part of their role, will be protected through the adoption of a 'professional persona' from thoughts and feelings which might otherwise damage their psychological well-being. Tasks such as the protection and removal of vulnerable people from close relatives, undertaking caring or tending which breaches normal codes of intimacy, such as medical examination, incontinence care or the handling of dead bodies, extract an emotional cost which the professional persona largely mitigates. Similarly, it may be necessary for an older person to adopt a certain persona, such as being entirely dependent or independent, playing dumb or becoming overly persistent and repetitive to be recognized, to gain a voice in age-stereotyped situations. Such performances gain what is required from a situation with minimal investment and protect the core self from potentially damaging exchange. They are, that is, a form of resistance to frightening or demeaning situations, as long as contact is restricted to short episodes or the protective function is robust and well rehearsed.

Within traditional understandings of analytical psychology, the persona is seen as restricting processes of individuation throughout the first half of life and is then effectively shed as individuation gathers pace in the second. This posture can now be seen to underplay two elements of the masking process. First, as has been pointed out by Brooke (1991), more parts of the self do not simply become available to consciousness as individuals mature: awareness of personal identity also becomes increasingly more abstract. This implies that the conscious ego is increasingly capable of reflexivity, becomes aware of differing aspects of identity and, by degrees, can influence their relative power at any one time. Second, an exclusive focus on individuation fails to recognize this protective role of the persona, emphasizing instead its inhibiting function. However, it is now argued that the social mask not only restricts self-expression, but also protects parts of the self that are vulnerable to social forms of attack. Once it is recognized that later life is also a period in which significant social constraints are placed on self-expression, the importance of a continued role for social masking as protection becomes clear.

In this context lessons can be drawn from Hopcke's (1995) observations on the use of persona-like resistances by oppressed or minority groups.

Older adults, while not referred to directly, would qualify as such a marginalized and stigmatized group. He argues that social marginality places gays, lesbians and people of colour in an ambivalent relationship with the persona, which becomes simultaneously a means of expression, of communication and of performance of an otherwise hidden identity and an expression of its denial. For 'social outsiders', Hopcke (1995: 13) claims, the persona performs an especially important function as a 'mask that feigns individuality'. Interaction between the persona and those shadow parts of the self that have to be denied in conventional social interaction is a contradiction from which a more complete sense of selfhood must come.

If resistance is centred on 'race', the problem becomes, according to Hopcke, one of invisibility in a dominant and potentially hostile culture. Conformity takes the form of unflattering caricature and individuals are placed in a double bind in which voice is achieved through a rejection of cultural rootedness. Lury (1996) has similarly described a tension between imitation and authenticity as being focal in exchanges between dominant and minority cultures. Under such conditions, accommodations to a dominant culture convey 'a pernicious sense of being an impostor, of not having deserved this status, of having fooled someone or gotten ahead unfairly.' Similarly, 'To capitulate to outsiderhood means a suppression of the self through persona falsification or identification, but to challenge outsiderhood may result in the development of a persona which in its authenticity is a threat to the stereotype and is therefore used to further attack and suppress the individual' (Hopcke 1995: 109).

As a gay man, Hopcke sees a solution in the display of previously hidden identities through masquerade, in which the mask becomes a channel for a sort of expressive liberation from everyday constraint. This parallels observations by Kaminsky (1993: 261) that marginalized groups need to create their own definitional ceremonies when faced with 'crises of invisibility'. Among Yiddish-speaking older people such ceremonies pose 'strategies that provide opportunities for being seen, and in one's own terms, garnering witnesses to one's own worth, vitality and being.'

Hopcke pushes the theoretical limits of persona, however, by claiming that there are authentic and inauthentic uses that can be made of it, which he identifies with the expression of increased individuation. A conventional Jungian interpretation of such a performance, however, would emphasize its regressive character as the restoration of a different, if more comfortable, mask, rather than a genuine expression of selfhood. The criticism is based on a presumption not that the expression of gayness is in some way regressed, but that masquerade is still an ingenuine way of expressing it. As a mechanism of transformation, Hopcke (1995: 210) claims that the mask 'eliminates the wearer's identity', thereby 'eliminating the ordinary self and liberating the wearer from everyday constraints so as to permit an expansion of self and a sense of freedom.' What this interpretation makes explicit is that personae can become a vehicle for the transcendent. And through the experience of 'identity reversals' the persona absorbs the impacts of wounding social stereotyping and, under certain circumstances, turns them against stifling conformity.

A discussion of changing patterns of social relationships in later life, of masquerade and of social personae has raised a number of questions that suggest a particular dynamic to the maintenance of an ageing identity. This dynamic will be explored in more detail below. The phraseology of persona and masquerade also requires elaboration at this point. Persona seems to imply episodes in which a relatively fixed identity is installed and deployed, while masquerade connotes a more dynamic process of performance which is undercut by external orders of control. One implies an inwardly driven deployment of identity, the other a more fluid response to social demands; one position, the other process. To express this amalgam of fixity and mutability, the term masque will be used. Masque refers to the arena of inner and external contingencies within which the deployment of personae and the performance of masquerade are contained.

THE MASQUE AND MATURITY

The concept of masque, which draws on persona and masquerade, can be used to elaborate two themes emerging as key to the management of a mature identity. First, there is a need to negotiate multiplicity, in terms of a wide variety of unstable social situations that arise through contemporary relations and in terms of the options available in the way that the self presents an acceptable face to others. Second, there is a need for cohesion and continuity which comes to light in the putting together of a personal narrative in the here and now and in grounding present experience of self in a personal past as a sort of pathway to the present. These twin requirements lend shape to contemporary forms that a mature imagination might take. In a modern context, maturity, particularly in later life, contains the contradiction that at the same time that a wide variety of opportunities for psychological development become available, creating inner sophistication, social expectation provides a series of increasingly marginal and restrictive social roles. The advent of postmodern conditions has made a plethora of identities available. However, these appear to be drained of significance and easily become a means of avoiding an encounter with existential questions of ageing. Both readings suggest psychological processes that at one level allow engagement with social expectation, whether multiple or restrictive, and at another protect personal coherence and continuing personal development.

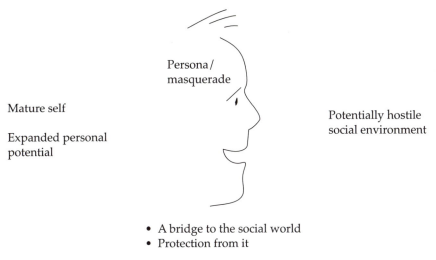

Persona/
masquerade

Mature self

Expanded personal
potential

Potentially hostile
social environment

- A bridge to the social world
- Protection from it

Figure 4.1   The uses of persona.

A logic for age-identity as protective strategy and as performance follows from these circumstances. It is concluded from what evidence on the subjectivity of mature adulthood and old age is available that there exists an experiential sophistication in maturity. Experience has made a variety of presentations of identity, a repertoire, available to the performer that was less available to earlier life phases, where deployment was either too inflexible or insufficiently varied in resources. This would suggest that the attribution of rigidity to the mature personality in ageist society is largely a projection, and an intolerant one, from a dominant and younger group. By contrast, a reading of age as increasing sophistication in the deployment of masquerade and movement between different priorities for the self may be particularly suited to the flexibility and contingency of identity required by contemporary society.

According to this viewpoint, and contrary to popular assumptions about the ageing process, maturity gives rise to an expanded capacity for self-experience. Rather than being primarily outwardly directed, it is directed inward as part of a 'duty to pay serious attention' to the self as a psychologically distinct, developing and spiritual entity. In addition to being something of a natural process in later life, this focus on internal coherence acts as an antidote to ageist ascriptions circulating in the social world. In order to survive, however, this process of becoming also requires shielding from notions of correct or 'successful' ageing imposed by a social milieu, largely hostile to the mature project of increased depth and self exploration, replacing it by expression through the mechanisms of restriction or surface multiplicity. This interpretation of the uses of social masking is shown in Figure 4.1.

An inhospitable social climate has made the deployment of protective identities an effective strategy and point of resistance against such predations of the self and also a means of ensuring continued self-development. In the inimicable spaces provided by a youth-obsessed culture, hospitals, surgeries, centres of social care, soap operas, supermarket checkouts and any number of the anonymized intergenerational encounters of everyday life, masquerade provides a way of keeping it simple. The real business of continued self-development can continue, unintruded upon, within. Masque, as an interaction of appearance and depth, has been made a necessity by changed life priorities that do not fit well with the age-ascriptions of the dominant culture; self-development by subterfuge against the ground of inhospitable constructions of age.

The functions required by a mature psyche are, then, to negotiate possibilities that emerge for self-presentation while maintaining a personal sense of coherence. This suggests the possibility of personal becoming at different levels and in the service of different psychological functions. At the level of persona and masquerade, the postmodern facility of mutation and multiplicity is preserved. The social mask, as the outermost layer of the psyche, acts to find a place in the social world through a delicate interplay of conformity to the expectations of others and the protection of personal thoughts and feelings from observation and interrogation. As such it contains that certain form of becoming which absorbs the props and opportunities, the episodes that facilitate the creation of a variety of identity statements. It becomes the surface on which identities are created.

At a deeper level of becoming, the psychological processes are organized around a guiding principle of personal coherence. Here, a sensibility for continuing self-development is maintained, of a different order from that arising from consumer culture and which approximates individuation and gerotranscendence. Masking and masquerade raises the question of what lies behind the masque and mature imagination, which, according to this view, is not a simple question of a perpetual interplay of surfaces. Rather, a masque intimates an entity behind the conceit and thereby a purpose to the patterning of masks and identities. This hidden intelligence resists the pull of the market-place of consumer identity. It emphasizes the interplay of self-continuity, cohesion and coherence within mature consciousness, in which memory is valued and experience built upon as the palate of an actualising self. Deeper still may lie an unconscious, personal or collective, the mindfulness or life-force that drives continuing self-development. The depth of identity conveyed here does not, however, intend a fixed series of psychological levels. It might, instead, describe distinctions that can be made in the process of negotiating connection between the social and the personal and that are the products of particular social and historical circumstances. It is suggested that the psyche coheres certain formations as various forms of threat and opportunity are encountered, and as part of that encounter the psyche becomes layered. Each layer holds, for a certain time, an amalgam of fixity and becoming, which, given other circumstances, may itself change.

LIKELIHOOD AND THE LAYERING OF MATURE IMAGINATION

This distinction between persona and masquerade as one layering of psychological process and a deeper project of personal coherence as another, makes available a psychological distance, an emergent containing space in which it is possible to think, reflect and experiment with the performative. A degree of choice is thereby allowed to enter performance, so that at times an identity may be created or adopted, but at other times the whole performative stance might be dropped. This latter attitude refers to a 'What the hell' response, of wearing purple hats, of an uninhibited display of self, regardless of the gaze of the other. This does not preclude occasions where a mature imagination can 'play' at being uninhibited, which is certainly a performative possibility. It indicates that the mature self is capable of using or discarding the performance of identity depending on circumstance or pure bloody-minded caprice. For most of the time, however, the space between personal coherence and masquerade centres on the likelihood of a performance being convincing. 'Likelihood' that a mask will sufficiently shield or disguise, that performance completes the bridge between the social and the personal, becomes a core organizing principle of identity in mature adulthood. How likely is it that I have to repeat myself to be listened to, how likely that I have to play at becoming dependent/independent to get my immediate needs addressed, how likely that I can appear ageless, youthful, wise, gracious?

Sometimes mask and self may be sufficiently compatible for underlying priorities and coherences to emerge through the mask; the mask becomes an elastic skin that enhances self-expression. At times this relationship becomes rigid and restrictive and at yet others the relationship is ambivalent, as it both hides and through the act of hiding reveals that something is being disguised. On occasions when the possibility of acting-through the masque arises, a degree of fit may be obtained between the mask adopted and the inner self. When this occurs, the expression of genuine experiences of ageing and the existential questions that ride in their train becomes a possibility. In circumstances inhospitable to the display of a mature and embodied identity, the mask worn would serve a protective function, a retreat into superficiality, whereby a state of unquestioning everydayness or parody might occur. However, these protections are deployed rather than becoming substitutes for mature identity. Indeed, it would be a signature of mature identity, should deployment following a deeper logic be taking place.

Questions of likelihood remind us of the connective function of the persona and that personal identity needs to be grounded in social relations in some form. This includes an attendant tension between selfhood as intersubjectively real and as internally coherent. Erikson, it has been argued, chose the first of these routes to self-expression, while Jung took the second. However, it is becoming increasingly clear that elements of both become apparent as ageing takes place. Both of these original formulations eclipsed the employment of masking, through either confounding mask and identity or negating its value. Both, alone, are inadequate to the task of negotiating a sustainable sense of selfhood. If the self were to become unconnected from the social, as suggested by a quest for a personal internal logic, then the possibility of distinguishing between fantasy and external reality would become diminished, if not impossible. Too exclusive a focus on the intersubjectively real, to see oneself as others see you, on the other hand, abjures those personal sources of coherence in favour of shifting social sand. In mature adulthood, forms of connectedness include embodiedness and its associated awareness of finitude, personal memory as well as social interaction. An exploration of masking as a communication between internal coherence and intersubjective meaning reveals that self-expression is both multilayered and multifunctioned. It is simultaneously a bridge between inner and outer worlds, can exact a toll of conformity, protects self-development in inhospitable circumstances, displays as well as hides the mature identity yet does not rupture the relationship between the personal and the social.

SUMMARY AND IMPLICATIONS

If the proposals for the mature imagination outlined here are accepted then certain conclusions follow concerning its subjectivity and shape. The subjectivity of mature adulthood is presented as being multilayered and in a dynamic relationship to the social conditions in which it is found. This layering supplies a connective yet protective function in relation to social reality, with different contexts supplying different possibilities for authentic self-expression. When these possibilities are restricted, either through negative stereotyping or a denial of ageing through multiplicity, mature subjectivity takes on a Machiavellian aspect. Authentic aspirations and potentials, which refer equally to de Beauvoir's projects and reflections on the 'real self' in the psychotherapies, are protected and subject to subterfuge. They exist at depth and reflect a need for coherence, occasioning a layering of the personality. Remembered experience and continuity of identity would be one source of integrity that is so shielded. When possibilities for the expression of an underlying selfhood are enhanced, masque becomes a flexible medium for communication, as internal and surface patternings of identity coexist and covary. They dance together in a marriage of fixity and change and a harmonious relationship between continuity and immediate coherence. According to this perspective, contemporary ageing is a process that can yield significant personal development, but rarely under circumstances of its own choosing. It is a process that requires strategies for positive maintenance and a balance between inwardly and outwardly directed personal development.

5

Midlifestyle

MIDLIFE AND THE MATURE IMAGINATION

Midlife has become an important cultural crossroads for the mature identity, bringing into sharper focus a debate on the relationship between appearance and authenticity. Should lifestyles developed in middle age be extended for as long as possible across the remaining lifecourse? Should midlife occasion a significant, and in some cases traumatic, break with the priorities of younger adulthood? Is it the case that midlifestyles have become an age-specified masquerade?

There is perhaps a tacit wish within the development of midlifestyles that the problems of ageing can be, if not eliminated, postponed almost indefinitely. This unstated desire is buoyed up by a wide variety of social currents, which include a move towards immediacy in psychotherapy and counselling, but also extend to include the representation of adult ageing in the media and in the production of midlife manuals.

One idea that recurs in the literature on mature adulthood is the notion that the cornerstones for a fruitful late life are set in the middle years. This is a trend which crosses disciplines and subject areas. In terms of economy, Cutler (1997) reviews an international policy concern about the readiness of midlifers to accrue resources, in terms of both disposable finance and independent lifestyles that will sustain them in later years. Erikson and his followers (1986), as has been seen, place significant emphasis on midlife generativity as a preparation for and determinant of psychological integrity in old age. Warnes *et al.* (1998) review the importance of healthy lifestyles adopted at this stage of life if health status is to be maintained in later years.

A reading of the literature on midlife is suggestive of at least two ways of interpreting the value of this period for the mature imagination. On the one hand, it is viewed as a distinctive episode in the lifecourse, in which certain questions about meaning and existence require a response. This perspective is closely allied to the idea that midlife provokes some form of crisis which itself marks a transition into a new phase of development. On the other hand, midlife has come to characterize a form of lifestyle in itself. This notion, of what has been called midlifestylism, includes within it a series of distinctive values and attitudes. Midlife is not portrayed as a point of lifecourse change, it is not liminal, in the sense that the first interpretation implies; rather, it marks a plateau which the successful midlifestylist maintains for as long as body, money and psychology allow. In both interpretations there is a tension between what can be chosen and what forces itself on to social, psychological and physical agendas regardless of the wishes of the individual.

The notion of midlife is therefore rich in paradox. It is marked by an awareness of increasing certainty in the lifecourse and of increasing uncertainty. The certainties include a growing apprehension of finitude, that things cannot go on for ever and that there is not an infinite amount of time in which to achieve all that one wishes in life. Time begins to take its toll, both as the generation above begin to die and as the effects of physical ageing etch themselves on to the personal body and those of one's contemporaries. At the same time these intimations of limit also increase awareness of the uncertain nature of existence. At a personal level they hold within them a narcissistic threat to one's own immortality, an increased anxiety and the beginnings of a search for a solution to this puzzling limitation on what had previously seemed to be an unending ascent. These new concerns may come to replace achievement anxiety associated with the building of a career and family. Indeed, normative expectations from the first half of adult life can take on a coercive quality if they no longer appear to fit newly emerging life goals and circumstances. A confusing patterning of social and physical life events begins to take shape during this part of the lifecourse. Midlife is a period of peak achievement and competence in many areas, yet at the same time it intimates that pre-existing goals and priorities may not hold. Unless alternative trajectories are explored, the future simply consists of a progressive narrowing down, in which doors are closing and on occasion are being closed unnecessarily by social structuration and interpersonal expectation.

While there are dominant trends, these may be mitigated by local and contemporary patterns. An increase in non-lifecourse determined mortality, such as that created by the AIDS epidemic, war or dramatic environmental change, might affect attitudes to mortality and serve to loosen the association between old age and death. Similarly, the spread of diverse lifestyles that do not necessarily conform to the standard model of the heterosexual, the nuclear and the work-determined might disrupt conventional conceptions of lifecourse development. Whatever the local forms are that affect the lifecourse, the disruptive influence of finitude adds a key source of indeterminacy to existing assumptions, plans and desires that had previously been assumed to be of unlimited duration. A second source of indeterminacy is added by the multiple options made available through consumer lifestyles. The consumer stance appears at one and the same time to gloss over intimations of finitude and, through its close association with identity as a form of masquerade, make them a covert focus of attention. Midlife itself might occasion a change from consumption as a means to further achievement, pleasure and self-enhancement, to consumption as a means of distraction, avoidance and diversion. From this standpoint, it appears that a modern privileging of the priorities from first-half adulthood and the siren call of postmodern lifestylism have strikingly similar conceptions of mature adulthood. These serve to highlight youth, agelessness and a fantasy that life goes on for ever, while other questions intrinsic to midlife and beyond are simultaneously made opaque.

MIDLIFE AND MASQUE

A key question arising from the discussion on masque and masquerade in mature adulthood would be how to construct an appropriate identity that at one and the same time protects a maturing imagination and maintains a form of connection to immediate social milieux. It raises a number of issues about the strategies used to balance these priorities, which would include the social spaces that can contain certain meanings for mature adulthood and the variety of options and social and cultural props available to maintain identity. Social spaces act as a legitimizing force to lend the lifecourse shape and definition, they are the scripts that a mature identity can read itself into. Conceptions of midlife may vary the scope available for the interplay between deeper, more enduring, more agentic aspects of the self and socially validated surfaces such as the persona and the masquerade. Insofar as midlife issues pertain to outer layerings of the psyche, they concern the construction of cohesive and flexible surfaces that depend for the most part on becoming intersubjectively real. Their coherence is focused more upon the degree to which they convincingly contribute to social episodes and statements of lifestyle than upon deeper forms of personal integration.

At certain points these constructions must have a touchstone to some other form of the real than their own logic; otherwise they risk spiralling off into self-contained and almost psychotic states. Grounding may come in the form of memory, embodiedness, continuity or community with others. However, in midlife the use of these forms is generally partial and in the service of fuelling a current narrative rather than exploring the authenticity of those sources in themselves. It is not necessarily the case, then, that one is told what mature adulthood is really like; rather, one explores a masque that is being played out.

It appears that a variety of scripts have become culturally available, which support certain interpretations of what midlife is about. Thus, midlife has been construed as a period of crisis, of transition, as a plateau which is maintained thenceforth, as resonant of other life phases. It is a construction, in other words, that emerges through certain discourses on the lifecourse, is mutable and not a biophysical fact of life. Social and biological events, such as menopause, sexual behaviour, redundancy, new careers, changes of partner or intergenerational commitments, are given emphasis and meaning depending on the reading of a particular midlife script.

MIDLIFE AS CRISIS

Within the Western cultural and scholarly tradition midlife has characteristically been seen as provoking some form of crisis of identity. Neugarten's (1968) early discussion of the appropriateness of life events included the view that people were 'clocking themselves' in relation to accepted, and largely unquestioned, life stages and rites of passage. The timeliness of life events referred to whether they occurred at the point in the lifecourse where majority behaviour would predict. Thus an adult who did not get educated, get married, have children, get a job at approximately the same age and in the same order as most of his or her contemporaries would be judged to be out of time, out of synchrony with the age cohort. Being on time or out of time with the accepted structure became a criterion for subjective satisfaction and socially valued norms of conformity.

Neugarten draws attention to a paradox in these cohort values and attitudes, which also mark a certain socio-historical positioning of midlife. In the 1960s, 'Middle aged men and women, while they by no means regard themselves as being in command of all they survey, nevertheless recognise that they constitute the powerful age group *vis-à-vis* other age groups; that they are the norm-bearers and the decision-makers; and they live in a society that while it may be oriented toward youth, is controlled by the middle-aged' (Neugarten 1968: 93). The middle aged, then, were in control, but within a society that was in the process of coming to terms with a burgeoning youth culture. They bore the norms that were about to come under sustained attack from that younger generation. The triggers for crisis among a group used to dominance were conceived as being biological (Brim 1974) in origin and as a consequence of work performance (Farrell 1975). As such, Western conceptions of midlife caught individuals out of sympathy with the general expectations of their society, yet this itself was to be expected as an inevitable product of that particular social construction of the lifecourse. This interpretation of midlife as crisis had its basis in functionalist social theories, whereby it was proposed that roles and relationships served to integrate individual aspirations into the wider social good, as reflected in pre-existing social structures.

Within the intellectual atmosphere of the 1950s and 1960s, midlife characterized a period that was both to be expected and in some way anti-normative. Social structuration around work and family made midlife a turning point, which developed an aura of crisis because it also required a shedding of dominant sources of self-worth. It could be said that midlife split the functionalist atom, insofar as it peeled social expectation off from individual desire and aspiration. It characterized a period of the lifecourse marked by an increasing lack of fit. The midlife adult was caught in a double bind, in which one could only become a good, age-normative citizen by acting out an individual resistance to social expectation. Midlife adults were expected to give up on the values that had previously served them well and seemed to be the only positive set of lifecourse values around. The normative expectation was thus one of initial resistance to narratives of disengagement and decline (Cumming and Henry 1961), to which the individual eventually succumbed and thereby got back into synchrony with what society expected of a man or woman of that age. It became a period of anticipated resistance, resolved for the greater functional good of intergenerational succession.

It is perhaps unsurprising that the notion of midlife itself, and of midlife as a critical lifecourse event, generated a simultaneous interest from writers in the psychodynamic tradition. Jaques (1965), who placed crises as occurring between 35 and 65 years, was at first interested in changes to creative, and most notably artistic, production. He described mature creativity as a development beyond the 'hot from the fire' approach of younger adulthood, towards a process of interplay, in which intuitive influences from the unconscious are combined with a considered apperception of a product and reactions to it. He then used psychodynamic case material to examine the depth psychology of this process and how it 'manifests itself in some form in everyone' (Jaques 1965: 506).

'The paradox is', he claimed, 'that of entering the prime of life, the stage of fulfilment, but at the same time the prime and fulfilment are dated. Death lies beyond.' This dual apprehension is exemplified in a remark from Jaques's patient, who observed that while one has gained the crest of the hill, and can now see beyond the upward slope, one can also see that the journey has to end. Jaques made his study of creativity and clinical material fit together by bringing Kleinian theoretical concepts to bear. He particularly focused on explanations of adult psychological processes in terms of an emerging 'depressive position', first encountered in early childhood development and re-experienced as a characteristic adaptive response to ambiguity throughout life. Somehow losses experienced by the infant, and in adulthood the awareness of personal death, had to be integrated into an individual's view of the world. The emergence of a depressive position does not mean, according to this view, that one gets depressed, but that one has managed to integrate both positive and negative experiences, and can hold them in mind at the same time. Death and the midlife crisis are intimately linked because they trigger the emergence of a new way of combining conscious and unconscious material that would otherwise be split off and lead to a fragmented personal identity. Accordingly, the crisis is an internal, existential one, which, if successfully resolved, results in what could be described as a more considered, integrated, yet melancholy state of being.

The influence of a psychodynamic approach can also be felt in cross-cultural studies that have expanded upon Jungian notions of difference between the first and second halves of life, and employed the distinctly psychodynamic Thematic Apperception Test. This test was designed to capture psychological projections by noting the associations respondents made to a series of drawings whose meaning was deliberately ambiguous. In particular, in Guttman's studies (Neugarten and Guttman 1968; Guttman 1975), midlife came to be seen as a period in which traditional, and most notably gendered, characteristics are reversed. Guttman indicates that in the second half of adult life women become increasingly engaged with life beyond the domestic, are more assertive, outward looking and socially dominant. Men, however, come to relinquish goals of social achievement and external agency and exhibit increased interest in caring, relationships, spirituality and 'magical mastery' through inner growth. These studies do not seriously question the gendered division of labour in younger adulthood. It is assumed that these tendencies towards child-rearing among younger women and work among men emerge as a response to what Guttman calls the 'parental emergency'. Once the child-rearing phase of the lifecourse has been completed, women and men have the opportunity to develop those skills that they had previously neglected. It is, perhaps, a specific interpretation of the analytic concept of individuation, but it is unclear what influence a historical blurring of rigid gender activities would have on such narratives of reversal.

King (1974, 1980) identified many of the issues associated with midlife for both genders as being problems of narcissism. She describes this as consisting of an 'Overvaluation of the self, inability to cathect their sexual partners with object-libido, who were treated as extensions of themselves, [such that] the actual needs of their objects were treated with indifference' (King 1974: 31). In other words, midlife is seen as a time of self-obsessed regard, with little thought or feeling for the effects of personal conduct on others. It is as if the midlife personality wanders, staring into a hand-mirror, through relationships made superficial and a future made unseen. Her patients rarely sought treatment directly because of these issues, however, as they were mostly concerned with the non-compliance of others to their will and otherwise 'were not aware of their ailment' (King 1974: 32).

King's explanation for the phenomenology of midlife that she describes rests on parallels between the developmental and psycho-social tasks posed during middle age and adolescence. The keynote here is that both are perceived as periods of transition, of 'sexual and biological change . . . exacerbated by role changes and their socio-economic circumstances' (King 1980: 156). Both lead to problems of activity and redundancy, dependency and independence, a change from two- to one-generation households and the making of new relationships, changes to self-perception and the perceptions of others. Cumulatively, these factors can precipitate a crisis of identity. The nature of these changes suggests that King is speaking about patients in later midlife, or those experiencing conflicts associated with associated age-norms. She indicates that resolution of these problems produces a similar broadening of psychological functioning to that described by Jaques.

The observation that people do not necessarily enter treatment to cope with a midlife crisis as such is repeated by Kleinberg (1995). He describes a 'character pathology' of middle age in terms that are not dissimilar to King's idea of self-absorption and the increasing staleness identified by analytic psychology. The pathology is described as consisting of: '1. The inability to enjoy sexuality; 2. The incapacity to relate in depth to other human beings, with lack of awareness of ambivalence and a lack of capacity for mourning over the aggression toward those who are loved; 3. A denial of aggression in self and others, expressed in naivete; and 4. The lack of a satisfactory, effective and potentially creative work situation' (Kleinberg 1995: 211). Kleinberg's interest lies in how this midlife dynamic is manifested in group situations. It is difficult, he argues, to voice these concerns in groups because of the risk of becoming a repository for the similar, yet projected and unaccepted feelings of other people in midlife. To admit concern in such a milieu is to admit weakness and carry the burden of that fear of weakness for others. Should such individuals participate in group therapy, Kleinberg argues, feelings of stagnation and frustration need to be worked through, even though a preoccupation with their own personal crises often makes it difficult for individual members to empathize with the similar concerns in the group as a whole.

There are also important differences between the management of identity in midlife and in adolescence. This may be particularly the case in the deployment of social masking. It will be recalled that for Erikson

(1982) the task of adolescence was to discover an acceptable adult identity. Finding, through repeated experiment, a preferred identity, a face that fits, came to be seen as the gatekeeper to entry to the adult world. Failure to do so would leave identity diffuse and unstable. The adolescent is seen as being able to adopt and cast off different social masks which protect an immature, tender and elusive self. Adolescence is marked by moods and enthusiasms, embarrassment and narcissism, as various personae are worn, slip and are replaced. While midlife also appears as a time of tension around identity and transition, it may be subject to a different dynamic (Biggs 1997c). In midlife the self is again presented with a choice of identities, but rather than being driven by external pressure to find an appropriate role, as was the case in adolescence, the midlifer discovers internal dissatisfaction with an identity that fits all too well. As midlife gains momentum, the building of a conforming identity, at considerable effort and psychic investment, is increasingly seen as a cost: 'Passion now changes her face and is called duty; I want becomes an inexorable I must, and the turnings of the pathway that once brought surprise and discovery become dulled by custom' (Jung 1967a: 331).

Reading Jung, it is possible to discern a series of responses to this dilemma, which come in and out of focus as the problem of identity is brought to the fore. At first the associations of younger adulthood are unquestioningly maintained as being 'eternally valid'. As dissatisfaction arises, the midlifer may cling to these existing certainties, attempting to perpetuate them in the face of disconfirmation from a variety of sources. Finally, as alternative potential becomes expressed, a more complete self is allowed into consciousness and a new, more rounded identity is found. This would lead to the conclusion that as social actors mature, the use made of social masking varies, from a rigid signifier of adopted roles to a more flexible use of the mask itself, the distanced use of multiple masking and in some cases the absence of masking altogether.

This interpretation of mask and identity at different life phases allows a personal history of masquerade to take shape. During adolescence, it would appear that there is considerable distance between the ego, 'the real me' as available to consciousness, and the masks adopted. However, each mask is inflexible: you either have it or you don't; in order to adapt, you cast it off and find another one. The glue, so to speak, is weak, while the alternatives are many. However, once a snug mask is found it becomes a fixed adult identity. According to this view, during the first half of adult life the glue gets stronger and stronger until this outer layer is indistinguishable from the self and one is in danger of becoming one's mask. At the same time the mask becomes more flexible with use, the tricks of social exchange more practised. The mask can be turned to many different situations, manipulated almost as if it were not a mask at all, just a plastic, and agreeably thicker, skin. Midlife then becomes a period in which the costs of masquerade are apprehended, and as mid-life develops, so does the mask as an irritant to the ego. It is less comfortable to wear, does not cover adequately, the glue has become hard with age; but it may be too painful to tear off. Samuels (1985) points out, for example, that removal brings with it the fear that the ego, previously protected, will disintegrate. Thus, an initial period, during which the individual becomes aware of this tension, may be marked by increased adherence to the mask and projection of unwanted personal attributes on to others, a period that would be dangerous to persons exhibiting the characteristics that are presently being denied in the self (Biggs 1989). It is only through the build-up of contradictions between the inner and outer worlds that distance is achieved and new identities are adopted. Eventually, psychological energy, which had been held in check by social conformity, is expressed in, Jungians would argue, a more fulfilling and holistic personality.

FROM CRISIS TO LIFESTYLE

The debate on midlife, as described above, merges two streams of discourse. One positions midlife in relation to social function and social exclusion, the other interprets it in relation to psychological change. A consequence of such a merger is a loosening of the antagonism between ideas of forward movement during the lifecourse and the notion of a continuation of existing themes. It may, in other words, be possible to progress by the adoption of a different set of priorities. A process has begun that problematizes linear development of the former sort and, in so doing, raises narratives of conflict and crisis. However, there is also a tension over the treatment of these descriptions of midlife as a recognizable, if socially constructed, experience. This tension concerns what should be expected in midlife, and what responses are to be considered adaptive. Should King's, Kleinberg's and Jaques's writings be taken to indicate that midlife gives rise to a number of attitudes and behaviours that could be explained in terms of a pathology, for example? Is it, as Jung (1967c) famously opined, that the person who clings to the priorities of a different, and in this case earlier, part of the lifecourse is suffering from some form of neurotic illness? Should the resolution of these tensions be to encourage conformity to an intersubjectively determined, if ageist, lifecourse pattern? Or is this concern over lifecourse direction itself a script, a narrative that can be adopted or not as the fancy takes us? Do people simply 'play' at having midlife crises as a handy way of explaining immediate concerns?

There is also a tendency in the above descriptions to domesticate midlife, to move from metaphors of crisis, rupture and resistance to ones of transition. Transition is more consensual, more mutative, a softer conception that opens the possibility of multiple options for mature identity. The debate, and thus the narrative of midlife, is moved on from a phenomenology of midlife anxieties to one of transmutation. Speaking in terms of transition opens the way for a different sort of discourse. It allows conceptions of adult identity to enter a Baudrillardized world of simulacra, popular culture and consumer fantasy where the transitory becomes an end in itself. If identity is continually in transit it is not fixed anywhere, and while the episodes and options available to it might be created intersubjectively, they avoid being grounded other than in a logic of their own. The possibility that particular age-based lifestyles present such an opportunity is a discussion to which we now turn.

MIDLIFESTYLISM

The issues raised in the previous section concerning the creation of narratives for midlife and beyond have been addressed by an academic and popular literature that has focused on an active construction of lifestyle. These lifestyles for maturity often do not maintain a clear association with ageing and the lifecourse, except as a point of negative reference. They are perhaps most marked by a sense of the continuous, that things can carry on very much on an even keel and without rupture, which at the same time appears to have been bleached of serious concern for continuity and the passage of time.

One manifestation of this process has been the extension of 'midlifestyles' of various sorts into later phases of ageing (Featherstone and Hepworth 1982, 1983; Conrad 1992), through, for example, the targeting of older consumers by advertising agencies (Sawchuk 1995). In purpose-built retirement communities (Kastenbaum 1993; Laws 1995) the material environment has been carefully designed to act as a prop to the performance of a simultaneously ageing and ageless identity. Such experiments have been famously described by the grey panther activist Maggie Kuhn (1977) as 'playpens for the old', their defining feature being an exclusion of communications and persons that might disrupt identities created within that protected space. Communes for older people as an alternative to traditional conceptions of late-life have been researched by Baars and Thomese (1994), as have 'snowbird' mobile communities by Mullins and Tucker (1988), each of which describes attempts by older adults to invent materially living environments that support particular lifestyles, with varying degrees of success.

Featherstone and Hepworth's (1983) seminal work on lifestyle was the first to identify a new attitude to middle age as celebrated in the popular media. They contrast the traditional image of middle age in UK newspaper cartoons of the 1970s and 1980s, including 'Andy Capp' and 'The

Gambols', with 'George and Lynne', who exemplify an entirely different lifestyle. The former characters have reference points that link them to notions of a traditional industrial working class and of an essentially conformist and lower middle-class protective environment, respectively, associated with norms and expectations of the immediate post-war period. 'George and Lynne' inhabit a somewhat different and narcissistic world of leisure and active sexuality, supported by George's unspecified executive position. Accordingly, this lifestyle allows 'individuals who look after their bodies and adopt a positive attitude toward life . . . to avoid the decline and negative effects of the ageing process and thereby prolong their capacity to enjoy to the full the benefits of consumer culture' (Featherstone and Hepworth 1983: 87).

George and Lynne have created their own environment in which to express their 'different' identity. When their age is mentioned within the cartoon dialogue, it is used as an opportunity for display and positive self-surveillance, in order to exemplify the characters' seeming immunity to the ageing process. Their differentness is expressed in comparison to the characters in rival newspapers, which the reader understands, and more explicitly to foils in their own strip. An exchange that illustrates this distinction takes place between Lynne and their neighbour, Alice. Whereas the svelte and eternally décolleté Lynne claims that 'life begins at forty', frumpy, traditional Alice states, 'But everything else starts to wear out, fall out or spread out.' By buying George and Lynne's paper readers are invited to identify vicariously with their midlifestylism and collude with the mockery of Alice's downward slope. Featherstone and Hepworth (1983) conclude that for such characters the good life is here and now and, as long as their protected world is maintained, they can continue to enjoy it 'deep into the middle years'.

The 1990s have seen midlifestylism become subject to a series of labels that attempt to describe, to fix, the increasingly indeterminate lifecourse. Sheehy (1996) has, for example, named emerging lifestyles as 'middlescence'. The 1997 edition of the *Oxford English Dictionary* catalogues two novel descriptions for the adult lifecourse as adultescence or middle youth, in other words a 35–45-year-old with interests typically associated with youth culture. Each demonstrates a broader trend towards the blurring of traditional life stages and an associated desire to name and segment it into ever reduced and fragmented elements. This tendency has been particularly salient, according to Holland (1996), in the expansion of adolescence, both to include ever younger children and spreading out into areas previously thought of as adult. Under the influence of consumerism, it appears that childhood has been peeled off from childlike and childish behaviour. It is thereby possible for adults to indulge in narcissistic enjoyment and spontaneity previously associated with childhood, while at the same time children are encouraged to feed off adult tastes. In

Holland's words, a 'dual audience of infantilised adults and precocious children' has been brought into existence by contemporary media and consumer culture. Such a process is perhaps more salient in adolescence because it is a cultural focus in Western societies.

The cultural flexibility associated with youth is also reflected in language, so that suffixes attached to the stem 'child', such as -hood, -like and -ish, have few counterparts during midlife and beyond. It may therefore be more difficult to give voice to the unpeeling of identities in maturity. Indeed, the language of maturity, middle age and old age lends itself to single and fixed positions rather than to multiplicity. Rather than describe the fluidity of midlifestyle as a series of interwoven trends, intimately associated with the passage of time, there is a tendency to see it as in some way fixed and immobile once it has been adopted.

Paradox is heaped on paradox once the variety of images made available by contemporary cultural environments is taken into account. The linguistic fixity noted above requires reconciliation with a multiplicity of material from consumer culture. Each image contributes an episode that could be employed as a prop for positioning the self in relation to age and in the creation of a life-script. In addition to images of deprivation and disadvantage characteristic of modern portrayals of age in welfare policy (Townsend 1981) and the mass media (Hobman 1990) can now be added an excess of identities that play upon midlifestyle aspirations. These range from specialist magazines and travel clubs for active older people, through to the growth of ironic satire in magazines such as the *The Oldie*. Age is deployed in a number of settings. Age as chic, in the use of older models by Issey Miyake in his 1995 'octogenarian collection'. Here we encounter older women as spritely, confident and sophisticated (*Guardian* 19 July 1997). Age as resistance, in an uneasy portrayal, verging on difference as grotesque, in the performance of theatre troupes such as DV8. Here we find a naked 70-year-old woman (the dancer Diana Payne-Myers) performing to subvert the rigid aesthetic norms of ballet, but placed in a piece along with an 'anorak wearing nerd', a shadowy voyeur and a young and disabled female dancer (*Independent* 27 July 1997). Age as pastiche, in the performances of the comic, Caroline Aherne, a younger woman who dresses as the prim 'Mrs Merton' and then subverts this persona by engaging in a series of salacious interviews with media personalities. Age as self-centred, as indicated in Diverse Productions' (1996) documentary on 'snowbird' lifestyles entitled *Spending the Kids' Inheritance*.

Most of these images have female subjects. Male identities appear less often and in less diversity. They conform more closely to the modernist pattern of threat and crisis. Male midlife is portrayed as a period of sudden and unpredictable change and periods of disruptive madness; of, as one wife, reported in the *East London Advertiser* (17 April 1997), put it, 'not playing with a full deck'. It is portrayed as a period of throwing up established work positions for second careers and the betrayal of longstanding relationships for new partners who are inevitably younger. It is portrayed, in other words, as prone to desperate experiment at a time of sexual and productive anxiety. In contrast to Mrs Merton, the most popular male comedy character of 1990s UK television has been Victor Meldrew, a rueful and resentful persona who characteristically creates the circumstances for his own downfall.

Typical of this novel and predominantly female accent on midlifestyle in the 1990s has been a flurry of interest in the 'mould-breaking' baby boomer generation as it reaches its fifties. These articles have a marked tendency to concentrate on the plight of ageing, and almost exclusively female, Hollywood stars as points of reference. Their tone is usually upbeat, noting that at 51 the British actress Helen Mirren had been voted sexiest woman on TV, and that Julie Christie, Jerry Hall and Meryl Streep 'still look terrific' and maintain a glamorous media career (*Guardian* 12 June 1997).

Ambivalence, when it is expressed, has been couched in the failure of the outside world to live up to expectation. The self-styled mould-breakers find around them a society that does not reflect the new world that they had hoped to build. This divergence is expressed in the language of age as 'the original founders of youth and pop culture felt that growing up was an undesirable option, not an inevitability' (*Independent* 1 June 1997) and now discover that it is happening to them. It is happening, one might say, to the generation who would not trust anyone over 30.

Within these articles, one finds a growing concern over the absence of a legitimate narrative for the second half of life: 'Everyone knows what young people are like: everyone knows what old people are like. What the hell are middle-aged people supposed to be like? I don't know the script, I don't know the play . . . all I know is that I am not yet decrepit enough for Mantovani but too long in the tooth for Nirvana' (*Guardian* 8 January 1996). An aggressive resentment at the immediate circumstances of midlife is expressed by the novelist Howard Jacobson (1998): 'We feel things closing down on us and yet, at the same time, we feel we've never been more powerful, intellectually, linguistically powerful. The idea of the young snapping at our heels with their twitching members and sexual prowess is nothing; we can have them for breakfast.'

Carlin (1996) undertook a series of journalistic interviews with Hollywood stars who are now in their seventies. Rather than finding a group who engaged in Baby-Jane like reclusiveness, he describes a number of ways in which people, steeped in a culture of youth and beauty, negotiated a mature identity. These identities appeared as their youthful media personae became untenable. Carlin's piece reads like a guidebook to the dilemma of negotiating a serviceable new identity beyond midlife:

how it is done in the belly of the media beast. His interviews describe a number of strategies. Some keep on going by taking their age cohort with them as an audience who know the original script, but can identify with the tricks of ageing. Age is portrayed in rueful guise and the star simultaneously distances herself from ageing itself, which is in some way happening to her and to which she supplies a commentary while continuing with her real role as entertainer. Others have persisted with the original conceit, playing, in various degrees of self-knowledge, the youthful mask. That the audience appears as interested in elements of the grotesque, of women in their seventies singing and dressing as teenage cheerleaders, as much as they are in the pieces being performed. This evidences a curious instance of denial on the part of the performers. Finally, there is an ironic stance, which locates the contemporary self within a social and historical process. The process of ageing and identity is perceived as subject to rapid changes in fashion, such as the switch from Marilyn Monroe as a feminine icon to those of the hippies and of flower-power naturalism, which these actresses experienced not only at first hand but at the eye of the storm. 'I'm too old to be beautiful and too beautiful to be old', says one respondent who has learned to laugh at her experience, yet at the same time build upon it. This last interview exhibits a toughness of spirit which simultaneously bears the scars of the struggle with youthful identity and has not entirely shaken it off.

NARRATIVE APPROACHES

For those who lead more everyday lives than the inhabitants of Hollywood, there is also a growing literature to help the ageing individual negotiate appropriate lifestyles amidst the paradoxes of simultaneously increasing determinacy and indeterminacy. Techniques are offered whereby identity can be serviced and recreated.

For Litvinoff (1997) an answer lies in 'life-coaching'. The USA, it is claimed, boasts around 3000 life coaches. The method promotes a feeling-based and individualistic can-do culture, which appears half counselling and half management consultation: 'A coach is a hybrid of business advisor, mentor, therapist, counsellor and grandma, who thinks you're perfect and wants you to be happy' (Litvinoff 1997: 4). Advice is often directive and can be delivered over the telephone 'for half an hour a week'. From this description, life coaching appears as an invigorating top-up, a five-minute management of the self.

A growing interest in the narrative elements of counselling and psychotherapy fits well with the servicing of midlifestyles and identities. This form of therapy would appear to contain many of the elements identified in previous chapters as characteristic in maintaining a postmodern identity. There is, for example, an emphasis on loosening the relationship between current identity and the personal and cultural past, a focus on creating appropriate identities in and for the here and now, an unpeeling of different aspects of the self and their recombination. It is a technology for reinventing the self which also adopts many of the elements of masquerade, of telling ourselves stories for maturity that can then be lived by. According to Feinstein (1997), mythic narratives are needed to address the 'large questions of existence', such as life, death and personal meaning. However, myths no longer remain stable for generations, and must now be personally recreated. Emphasis is placed on the production of a servicable continuous narrative rather than on continuity with a particular culture and past. Within a narrative approach, 'the task of the counsellor is viewed at that of assisting the client to "re-author" parts of the life story' (McLeod 1996: 173). The therapeutic process consists of the retelling of a life story and the construction of a new guiding narrative. There are no value judgements made about the relative validity of old and new narrative, except in terms of the client's satisfaction with the story that emerges. Counsellors such as Spence (1986) consider that historical truth should give way to 'narrative truth', which McLeod (1996: 175) describes as 'the construction of an account of events that is coherent and allows the client to live a satisfying life.' According to Rennie (1994), a narrative helps a client to maintain distance from an inner disturbance, while simultaneously allowing some covert processing of issues surrounding it.

McAdams (1993) is perhaps the best known exponent of the narrative tradition. He claims that 'Defining the self through myth may be seen as an ongoing act of psychological and social responsibility. Because our world can no longer tell us who we are and how we should live, we must figure it out on our own' (McAdams 1993: 35). McAdams (1985, 1993) has taken a particular interest in the construction of identity in midlife. This he conceives of as a time of 'putting it together'. The hallmark of a mature identity is perceived as 'integrating and making peace among conflicting imagoes in one's personal myth'. These imagoes are the alternative identities that McAdams believes are collected by people in their thirties and early forties. Midlife, which is seen as stretching from the forties to the late sixties, then consists of a massive sorting out of these accumulated aspects of self. According to McAdams, as individuals move through midlife they become preoccupied with their own myth's 'denouement', and become more tolerant of the contradictory quality of existence. This reorganization of life's material takes place, however, in the service of the present: 'When the present changes, the good historian may re-write the past – not to distort or conceal the truth, but to find one that better reflects the past in light of what is known in the present, and can reasonably be anticipated about the future' (McAdams 1993: 102).

In fashioning a history for the self, one becomes one's own mythmaker and is seen to move towards 'post-formal' and 'local' truths. According to this perspective, identity in midlife and beyond becomes a matter of 'situationally specific truths, on solutions and logical inferences that are linked to and defined by particular contexts' (McAdams 1993: 200). The narrative that McAdams and others have described is not a simple process. It includes elements of immediacy, of the here and now, which lead to identities that are pragmatically created to meet current needs. A postmodern emphasis on episodes and situations rather than continuities has been retained, as has an ability to reconstruct the self based on immediate personal concerns. However, there is a simultaneous awareness of processes and changes in self-perception that relate to the lifecourse as a whole. Narrative therapy describes a technology of the self which fits midlife well. It simultaneously recognizes and attempts to rewrite the lifecourse script.

MANUALS FOR MIDLIFE

The indeterminacy surrounding ageing as an identity has led to a number of manuals, which in their varied ways constitute an attempt to interpret the changing lifecourse. These manuals claim to map the changing phases of maturity and add definition to its shape, thereby reflexively creating a view of the lifecourse in their own image. Within them are a number of answers to the questions that mature identity raises, which range from the elimination of ageing to the now familiar territory of age as a reinvention of self. Three attempts to rechart the lifecourse are examined below.

In *The Middle-aged Rebel*, Peter Lambley (1995) states that at the time of writing he was 48 years old, had almost retained the fitness gained in his twenties and was several times happier than he was in young adulthood. He draws on the particular cohort experience of the post-war boomer or 'Woodstock' generation, who now find their customary attitude as critics of the status quo undercut by having themselves become something of a cultural establishment. The answer to midlife anxiety that Lambley proposes is to take up this challenge by learning how to 'rebel constructively and responsibly against traditional ideas'. This is achieved in a typically 'boomer' way of taking control of what is happening through diet, exercise and a process identified as 'dream-mapping'. Dream maps, it is argued, take shape between the end of childhood proper, identified at approximately six years old, and the onset of adolescence, and are themselves a subtle form of rebellion, although the precise nature of the object of this rebelliousness is unclear. Subsequent development through relationships and work includes attempts to flesh out the dreams, in the belief that, as Lambley claims, we 'had the power to get what we want'.

By midlife, these dreams have been undermined by a series of compromises. Once these compromises have been critically re-examined, it
will be discovered that the greatest hindrance to self-development is the
previous inability of the reviewer himself or herself to learn the art of
responsible rebellion. This process leads to a rediscovery of the personal
dream, adapted to the more complex environment of established relationships and obligations that is typical of the middle of the lifecourse.

The *Middle-aged Rebel* is marked by a continuity of style. The life
experience of the 'Woodstock' cohort, of increasing personal choice and
self-expression, is now applied to the puzzle of ageing. It is thus a
generation-specific response to midlife and bears the hallmarks of other
social problems and barriers that this cohort has seen itself as overcoming. There is little recognition of difficulty beyond the reach of increased
self-management, 'taking control' of relationships and personal health
care. Midlife rebels, who must now rebel responsibly, also appear to
have pushed the recognition of a similar period in the lifecourse back
from that identified with crisis. If there is a golden age to which the
dream map, rediscovered in middle age, refers, it appears not in a transition similar to adolescence, but in the pre-teen or latency period. If
adolescence was marked by crisis and confusion of identity, the search
for a secure adult persona and the taking up of responsibility, this is not
the case during latency. Latency, as the label suggests, is marked by an
absence of conflict. Latency is pre-sexual and characterized by sensations
of certainty and autonomy, where identity is not cast as problematic and
relationships with others are rapidly being outgrown.

A very different response to ageing can be found in a second manual:
Deepak Chopra's (1993) *Ageless Body, Timeless Mind: a Practical Alternative
to Growing Old*. Here the problems of ageing are addressed in a characteristic and, as its title suggests, iconoclastic manner. It is claimed, through
an amalgam of ideas including social constructionism, quantum physics
and traditional Hindu meditation and philosophy, that ageing is essentially illusory. The logic of this argument is approximately as follows. An
experience of ageless body and timeless mind can be achieved because
our notions of ageing are mental and social products and are therefore
mutable. Further, the link between mind and body is far greater than
Western dualism would suggest, a point which draws support from the
indeterminacy of substantive boundaries between objects and energies
discovered by contemporary physics. A link between the mutability of
social, psychological and physical ageing is thereby established within
the internal logic of Chopra's position. Meditation, in conjunction with
healthy eating and exercise, is proposed as an appropriate technology
with which to influence this mind–body continuum as ageing arises from
the experience of stress and a habitual reliance on interpretations rooted
in the past. These are thought to cause mutations in our molecular struc-

tures that lead to the breakdown and entropic decay of embodied/mental processes. Openness to immediate experience and acceptance of events as they unfold are pitted against a tendency to store feelings as a form of 'emotional debt'. Insofar as the former can be enhanced and the latter reduced, ageing can be progressively abolished. The reader is thereby invited to become a pioneer in a new country where death and old age cease to exist and are, it is claimed, not even entertained as possibilities.

According to this perspective, age can be eliminated through the maintenance of an eternal present. The argument is sustained through a blurring of previously discrete discourses, such as physics, health care and Eastern philosophy, a characteristic that some authors (Crook *et al.* 1992) have identified with postmodernity. The appropriate technology of the self is based on meditation. There is no golden age from which midlife gains its character, because age is, at root, a diversion. In this respect Chopra's manual also includes aspects that Katz (1996) has identified as a pre-modern attitude to age. Age is conceived not as a stage that each person has to go through, but rather as a state of being. Wisdom, for example, can be a property of extraordinary people such as Jesus or Gotama, the Bodhisattva, regardless of their chronological age. There is little room in this perspective for an apprehension of personal history and continuity, which are seen as emotional debts clogging up the psychic economy.

Gail Sheehy's (1996) *New Passages: Mapping Your Life across Time* is perhaps the popular book most often cited in the human interest columns of broadsheet newspapers. It has been quoted in connection with 'boomer' activities, positive ageing and life counselling. She is cited (*Guardian* 4 January 1997) as deciding in her mid-fifties to reshape her body through jogging, yoga and aerobics, which she found to be empowering, and stating that others should follow suit by similarly 'reinventing themselves both physically and psychologically'. Sheehy postulates a new division of the adult lifecourse into provisional adulthood (18–30 years), followed by first (30–45) and second (45–85 plus) adulthoods. This later period is further broken down into an 'age of mastery' between 45 and 65 and an 'age of integrity' from 65 until death. Death itself is only alluded to, however. The rollcall of new age-stages continues on to include the sage seventies, uninhibited eighties, noble nineties and celebratory centenarians. And, while Sheehy cannot resist a gung-ho, can-do labelling of each adult decade (tryout twenties, turbulent thirties, flourishing forties, flaming fifties and serene sixties complete the set), her work includes a substantive attempt to reconcile cohort experience and the repeated challenges thrown up by the human life cycle. In so doing, she unpeels progress through various stages from the particular population characteristics and historical circumstances of any one group of adults. According to this view, each generation, identified by reference to the dominant political era in which it reached late teens/young adulthood, collects distinctive clusters of values which are then carried throughout the rest of adult life. However, it does greater justice to Sheehy's model if these values are thought of as something approaching guiding principles or core aspirations rather than fixed forms of behaviour. Fixity, as it appears in her 'new map of adult life', is an 'inner' experience that remains 'true to stage'. Sheehy's model would contextualize manuals such as Lambley's (1995) as an exemplar of one cohort's negotiation of the lifecourse.

Sheehy pays approximately equal attention to the contemporary lifecourse as experienced by men and women, from which women emerge as the most adaptive. In midlife, for example, Sheehy's pioneering and postwar 'liberated generation' of women appear to have gained in redefining their social relations. This is a group described as sleek, alcohol-free and successful in career, flicking through the pages of the best relationship guide. However, she is scathing of attempts to deny the existence of a biological clock and the expectation that medico-technical fixes can be found should motherhood have been postponed beyond peri-menopause. The menopause itself, however, should be planned, just as one plans pregnancy. Men of this generation, however, appear as ruefully contemplating a series of illusory vanities concerning sexual performance and economic failure. A solution is to be found in the 'sexual diamond', a recycling of Guttman's (1975, 1987) observations on role reversals in later life. Men, it appears, need to become connected to emotional intimacy with partners and offspring.

It is worth noting that this analysis also finds revitalization in a rediscovery of earlier life stages, and again parallels are drawn with preadolescence. Later life is marked by a rediscovery of 'zest'. This follows the passage through the biological and social menopause and, it is suggested, leads to a rediscovery of the 'wild girl's' feisty 'seeker-self' that existed before periods and other intimations of adult sexuality had begun.

While Sheehy's mapping of the adult lifecourse is upbeat and internally convincing, it is drawn from a relatively restricted social grouping. Her British examples almost exclusively emerge from dinner-party conversation and interviews with what might be historically located as 'New Labour' media professionals and executives. Her US sampling consists of a questionnaire survey of 'professional women and men', a *Family Circle* reader's panel and a survey published in *New Woman* magazine. While she is aware of the socio-economic bias that her samples include, this is justified because it is claimed that these groups break new ground and set new norms for her vision of an ageing lifestyle.

Sheehy associates 1990s midlife with mastery: this is identified as a process of psychological development of the self, rather than the socially sanctioned control that Neugarten identified in the 1950s and 1960s. She also identifies successful ageing as being resonant with other life phases, most notably pre-adolescence. She unpeels attitudes to ageing from cohort experience and identifies each cohort as having a particularized notion of what success in later life might mean. However, these notions are set in adolescence, reflecting her favourable citation of Erikson's model of identity formation. Their fixity within the lifecourse as described by Sheehy means that each of the challenges that the ageing individual must meet are interpreted within the framework of that particular and historically determined viewpoint.

MIDLIFESTYLE AS A SURFACE

Each of the manuals outlined above promotes a particular view of ageing and suggests strategies for midlife and beyond. They map out lifestyle narratives which place varying emphasis on the importance of the here and now, the role of experience, the possibilities for recombination and change. Chopra, for example, advocates the evacuation of the past and the tuning of consciousness to the immediate present. Lambley and Sheehy contain a mixture of exhortations including the continuation of strategies that have been learned at earlier phases of life, adapted to novel socio-cultural conditions. The latter two authors also locate a golden age, where autonomy was experienced and dream maps were formed, in pre-adolescence. This is strikingly different from the most approximate life stage chosen by a preceding cohort of writers, who had drawn parallels between transition and challenges to identity in adolescence and those occurring in midlife itself. It would seem that Featherstone and Hepworth's (1989) 'youthful self', hidden behind their mask of ageing, has now been given an age. However, in these manuals, it is an age of rediscovered expression, freed of the cares and responsibilities associated with adult identity. The manual writers describe mature adulthood in utopian terms. There is a shedding of old responsibilities and an opening of reconstructed, rediscovered and at the same time more authentic identity. It does not reflect the struggle with the body that is characteristic of postmodern theorizing on age, and neither does it reflect the elements of resistance to social stereotyping and personal fragmentation that can be found within the psychodynamic tradition. There is no place in these manuals for disconcertingly changed priorities or intimations of limit and mortality.

It was argued earlier that many of the questions surrounding midlife identity concerned social spaces that are created and maintained inter-subjectively and in which different versions of ageing could be played out. The formulation of midlife as crisis was, for example, rooted in a construction of old age that was intersubjectively real and related to issues of production and reproduction. Members of society tacitly agreed on a common-sense view of the mature lifecourse, the place of midlife rebellion and a pattern for an aged identity beyond it. The landscape was relatively fixed and the expected route mapped out. A paradox existed, in that people were expected to rebel against the next phase of adulthood even though the rebellion itself constituted a form of conformity.

In manuals for the new millenium, responsible rebellion has been transmuted into a means of continuing established patterns of identity management. There is little emphasis placed on the intersubjective insofar as it forms a glue for social relationships and agreed social meanings. It is clear, however, that the authors assume an almost self-evident rapport between their audience and their reconstructions of the lifecourse. Their reports are at some level believable.

What, then, is the intersubjective glue, the social understanding of what the world is like, that holds these narratives, these performances, together? First, there is a strong element of rejection of the traditional, age-staged, lifecourse. This is the element of rebellion. However, rather than moving on, either to a role with reduced status or to an increasingly individuated inner self, the map contains strong elements of cohesion around either a continuation of the present or the rediscovery of a golden age. Second, there is a marked absence of the social, both in the sense of relatedness to other people and in an unwillingness to include socio-economic factors that might facilitate or impede the adoption of a midlifestyle. This has been replaced by an individualized self, who may meet with like-minded others who themselves become props to the identity being constructed. Third, the manuals reflect the now familiar perspective that the personal past can be used to rebuild the self for current purposes, or under certain conditions should be rejected altogether. This position tends to evacuate personal history and continuity as contents of the self, although it appears that the manuals retain the continuous application of processes of self-presentation learned at other stages of the lifecourse. These points tend to reinforce adaptation to the essentially episodic and indeterminate social environments described by Giddens (1991) and Bauman (1995), and make the manuals an example of a postmodern technology of the self.

However, there is at least one area in which these manuals differ from the postmodern pattern. Each relies heavily on the power of personal agency, of an act of will that keeps a mature identity on the road. The problem is not seen to lie in the perceptions of others. For Hepworth (1991) the problem lay in the fact that the body is the symbol that external observers take to signify personal identity, and, as identity consists of an accretion of social discourses and attributions, influences negatively any sense of self. Thus, 'The self is only a looking glass self and as such is only accessible to us through the eyes of others' (Hepworth 1991: 96). For the 'pioneers' identified by Sheehy, Chopra and Lambley, this is not the issue. The issue is finding the personal will to reinvent oneself. And reinvent oneself in a way that still maintains the parts of the self which are wanted on the voyage.

So the intersubjective glue that binds the new midlife story together is, paradoxically, a denial of the intersubjective and a fetishization of an autonomous and self-creating self. Narrative approaches are valuable in this context because they supply the tools and an ideological justification for such an enterprise. They recognize the past while making it docile, subservient to current preoccupations and the creation of believable spaces in which to perform new identities. The identities which are created do not, however, appear to act primarily as a bridge to the social world, as was the case for the persona. They have adopted the protective role of the persona in the sense that midlife attitudes and strategies are sustained, but appear to have dropped its connective function to a wider social world. We are left with an internal construction about what midlifestyle might be in a social world, which has been substituted for a genuinely intersubjective and mutually constructed social environment. In this, the view of ageing, or of choosing not to age, as an act of will has taken on a life of its own.

SUMMARY AND IMPLICATIONS

This combination of attitudes to the past, the social and fixed age-expectations has led to a particular mutation of social masking and the relationship between the inner and outer psychological worlds. The protective performance of identity relies heavily on its own inner logic to stay cohesive and believable. Believability is largely defined in terms of the internal coherence of the stories that people tell themselves. Social connection is underplayed or used as a negative point of reference. This reliance on an inner logic for social conduct means that performances in social milieux can be believed to be true, while avoiding contact with possibly disturbing and disruptive external information. If this form of masquerade is typical at this life phase, then it constitutes a powerful means of negotiating the tension between increasing certainty and increasing uncertainty that characterizes midlife. In response to the uncertainties of contemporary living, one constructs a more certain personal narrative that holds social episodes and props to identity together within a cohesive storyline. This narrative may draw on existing social metaphors of crisis, transition or midlifestyle. Other sources of certainty are, however, less easily explained. Such strategies are achieved at a considerable long-term cost if their reliance on cohesion through the manipulation of surfaces and the likelihood that a particular narrative will be sustained fails to connect with the certainties of bodily change, a finite existence and deeper forms of psycho-social integration. At one level such strategies constitute a denial of ageing and things associated with it: value of memory, learning from experience, existential finitude. At another they constitute a practical strategy, given the resources to back it up. They are a step into the void left by the blurring of the lifecourse.

6

Meaning and forgetting

BEYOND MIDLIFESTYLE

While midlifestyle addresses the surfaces of identity, it begs the question of what lies beyond. The mature imagination must, in other words, maintain a convincing narrative of self in a continuous present and find a place for other, possibly more disturbing, aspects of the ageing self as well.

Mature identity has, then, to negotiate two principal processes, one which has been emphasized by broadly modernist interpreters of the lifecourse and another drawn from postmodern thinking. The modernists prioritize the view that while there is a drive towards the expansion of the self in later life, aspects that cannot be legitimately expressed are protected from an inhospitable environment. They are thus hidden from public view and in some instances from personal awareness. The psychodynamic approach to identity would be an example of this way of thinking. The postmodern interpretation emphasizes the negotiation of multiplicity and the opportunities that many different social constructions of identity can create. Later life consists of the construction of narratives which meet identity needs in the here and now, a process which is limited primarily by bodily ageing.

The view taken here is that both interpretations can be used to give shape to mature identity. People in maturity have, in other words, to negotiate multiple options for identity performance and find some way of dealing with aspects of their personality, and potential and existential needs, which cannot find expression in environments that are diverse yet are inevitably assumptive realities, with attendant opacities and taboos around ageing. Contemporary society appears to hold within it a capacity for ever-widening narrative sources for self-identity which are increasingly disembedded from their original contexts and attendant limitations. This can be seen in the changing interpretation of midlife from a period of crisis brought on by a lack of fit between personal desires and a fixed series of social expectations to a period of personal maintenance through continued midlifestylism. The history of an acceptable midlife has thus moved from using a metaphor of crisis to using one of transition and finally to self-narration. Midlifestylism, as the latest in this line, is dissimilar to other notions of personal renewal provoked at this point in the lifecourse, such as individuation (Jung 1933a) and gerotranscendence (Tornstam 1996). Individuation, for example, posits the development of characteristically different psychological processes and priorities beyond midlife from those that have dominated earlier life phases. A characteristic of the 'new' identities to be found in the midlife manuals and cultural identity statements outlined in Chapter 5 is their tendency to reconstitute the processes and priorities of earlier life phases to make sense of the demands of maturity itself. This may take the form of extending the life of strategies from younger adulthood to new challenges or drawing an analogy with a period prior to adulthood proper. While appearing to have similarities with the mainstream psychoanalytic preoccupation with the power of past, and in particular childhood events, such similarities are on closer examination superficial. A point of difference from psychoanalytic thinking is that the notion of a real and determining past has been ejected, in favour of a past that can be reinvented and used metaphorically. This works in favour of the continuation of patterns which, while harking back to, for example, pre-adolescence, do so in order to describe the continued use of stratagems and attitudes of the early–middle phases of adult life.

This kind of identity conforms to Bauman's description of a 'world in which the art of forgetting is an asset no less, if no more than the art of memorising, in which forgetting rather than learning is the condition of continuous fitness . . . boasting a lifelong guarantee only thanks to that wondrous ability of endless self-effacing' (Bauman 1997: 25).

An implication of Bauman's description of postmodern identity is that the experience of self approximates a videotape, rather than, for example, a family photo album. The former can be continually erased and recorded, whereas the latter is characteristically organized longitudinally and maintains images over time. Bauman argues that a casualty of the 'videotaping' approach to identity is that it breaks the link between cause and effect and in so doing insulates people from responsibility for their past actions. This he sees as a consequence of the episodic nature of contemporary culture. Viewed from a lifecourse and psychodynamic perspective, it could also be argued that active adoption of a lifestyle based on these premises supplies a mechanism for not connecting with personal causes and effects. It provides a mechanism for escaping the perception of existence as a temporal, longitudinal phenomenon, and the mortality that those trends would imply.

An additional characteristic of extended midlife can be identified in its focus on the power of a personal will, independent of social realities. Self-invention has become the socially agreed way of negotiating the lifecourse, yet one that simultaneously denies the fact that social agreement has anything to do with the process of recreating the self. In other words, the socially accepted common-sense that binds this narrative of self-creation together is paradoxically one that rests on eclipsing socially legitimized forms of identity as an explanation. The power of the social only really appears in a negative relationship to the self, in a rebellious stance against the fixed social construction of life stages. The inter-subjectively valid assumption that holds these views of social identity together is therefore based on a negative, a denial of their social nature and a denial of what is unacceptable to that newly created reality.

Taken together, these characteristics fill out a new legitimacy for mid-life and beyond: that the self can be continuously reinvented, in the process of which aspects of maturity that are negatively valued can be avoided. Social slights and contradictions need not form barriers to this self-contained project of personal invention. It is partly this process, with its elements of creative invention and self-deception, that makes the conflation of self and surface so difficult to distinguish in these identity statements and stories. They appear to be describing an expansive and liberating fulfilment of the self, while really only describing another form of social conformity. In appearing to deny the adoption of a social mask, they eclipse the ways in which the self has become mistaken for, has become for all intents and purposes, a masquerade. Identity and mas-querade inhabit the same conscious space and consequently selfhood appears as a series of surfaces, and, on first examination, that is all there is to it. The act of masking has largely lost its role as a bridge between inner and outer worlds. Instead, it is believed that a mature identity can somehow exist independently of social and ageing processes, even though it is the very existence of these processes that has made the masking necessary in the first place. The result is that midlifestyle subsists on its own internal logic and as long as that internal logic is not broken, it does not need to come into serious contact with realities that lie outside it.

Midlifestyle solves the problem posed by masquerade in the sense that content and purpose are supplied to the surface layering of the psyche. Its logic addresses the problem of how to tie the episodic and fragmentary processes of the social world into a cohesive narrative. It supplies, to paraphrase McAdams (1993), stories that can be lived by. It also provides a means of overcoming negative social stereotyping of later life associated with dependency and decline. The emphasis placed on personal will, narratives in the service of the present and control, denies such stereotypes a purchase on the new identities being created and recycled.

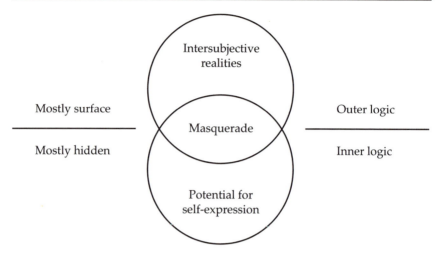

Figure 6.1   Hidden and surface logics.

Midlifestylism does not solve the problem of what lies behind the mask, however, as it is strongly bounded by its own terms of reference. The relationship to any deeper logic of the psyche is not addressed. It is trapped in a logic of its own making, beyond which it cannot see, and therefore lives within a constantly changing yet ever present sense of the immediate. Wider questions of lifecourse adaptation and change are avoided.

As ageing progresses, the psyche becomes layered in terms of the hidden and the surface in a particular way (see Figure 6.1). Some things become hidden and some surface because circumstances, the balance achieved between the internal logic of the masque and intersubjective reality, define what can and what cannot find a legitimate voice. What cannot be voiced gets hidden, but is not necessarily driven into the unconscious. Rather, it is possible that an outer layer can have one logic which is only tangentially related to the deeper internal logic of the psyche. This deeper logic contains possibilities for self-expression, which emerge as the lifecourse continues, but may be difficult to display publicly.

BEYOND SELF-NARRATION

There are a number of instances in the conception of ageing as self-narration that should give us pause for thought. First, there is a distinct resonance, a family resemblance, between the characteristics of the mid-life identity described in popular culture and life manuals, and those descriptions of narcissistic pathology found in the psychodynamic work of King (1980) and Kleinberg (1995). Both describe a preoccupation with the value of oneself as an individual, a devaluation of the social and of relatedness to others, plus a tendency to perceive others and the past as props in the service of immediate personal need.

Second, there is almost no mention of the two great contemporary fears associated with ageing, namely mental incapacity and bodily frailty. Although the prevalence of dementia, for example, which Kitwood (1997) estimates to be in the region of seven per cent for the population over 65, is low, it has come to dominate everyday fears associated with ageing. Dementia is in many ways a metaphor for the erosion of the mask, an inability to control or even remember the presentation of self for long periods. It is a process that requires grieving of social losses during periods of lucidity and active support in the maintenance of personal narrative (Cheston 1996; Mills 1997). In this sense it stands for the death of the masquerade project. The ageing body and its betrayals (Featherstone and Hepworth 1989; Turner 1995) has, as has been argued earlier, become a harbinger of postmodern despair. Both are disproportionately associated with adult ageing, yet neither features in the narratives of later life as a midlife extension.

Third, while proponents of the narrative approach, most notably McAdams (1993), have shown an interest in the creation of life-stories in mature adulthood, little is said beyond midlife narrative formations. In *The Stories We Live By*, for example, McAdams concludes with a three-page epilogue in which late-life issues are described as post-mythic. Eriksonian notions of integrity and life review are then employed to make sense of experience beyond the reach of midlifestyle. It would seem from this that the narratives, personae and masquerades arising in midlife cannot extend their reach indefinitely.

ALTERNATIVE LOGICS OF LATER LIFE

What might be the alternative logic for later life that is obscured by the masque of midlife narrative? What has been made taboo? What is hidden by the new orthodoxies? What fills out the deeper layers of the mature psyche? In many ways the hidden would represent the unacceptable, the shadow of the fantasy of continued midlifestyle. Where there is ageless-ness, there is also finitude. Where there is activity, there will be reflection. Where there is separation, there will be connection. Where there is paradox there will be integration. Where there is immediacy there will be attempts at coherence across the lifecourse.

Struggles to achieve a coherent psychology beneath the mask would include the apprehension of finitude and a simultaneous and growing awareness of connection. These twin concerns are not discrete: they inter-connect with the past and the future, merge and separate as part of a search for personal and wider social meaning. A concern with the finite nature of existence has been recognized in the writings of Jaques (1965), Jung (1931) and McAdams (1993). It rests on the acceptance that life will come to an end and that one must therefore begin to look forwards as well as backwards for reference points across the lifecourse. It is manifest in a growing curiosity concerning the denouement of one's own life story and refocuses attention on to sources of continuity. The ultimate destination for finitude is death, to which the bodily, mental and social losses associated with old age often act as premonitions. A concern with a connection to realities greater than the self is reflected in issues such as generativity (Erikson, 1982), spirituality (Tornstam 1996) and social connection (de Beauvoir 1970; Kuhn 1977). These processes of greater connection and personal closure also affect the perception of self, most particularly in the relationship between the past, the future and the present. As such they concern memory, death and sociability, each of which provides the potential for grounding personal experience and the lifecourse. In terms of personal phenomenology, or self-experience, these concerns translate into a process of looking backwards over the lifecourse to that which has already occurred, looking forwards to what has yet to happen and looking at sociability in the present.

CONTINUITY AND MEMORY

As we have seen, a core element within the psychoanalytic tradition consists of making sense of past life. This may take the form of uncovering memories that have been lost, which would serve to facilitate a release from the grip of unremembered and thereby unconscious power. It may take the form of obtaining a sense of order in the lifecourse, as suggested by adherents to ego psychology. In whatever guise it appears, memory has been placed in a central position in the process of becoming a more complete and self-directed individual. Memory has thus become the repository for unresolved contradictions and a source of material in using past life to understand contemporary identity. As such, it draws on powerful traditions within Enlightenment thought. It is the loss of memories beyond the possibility of retrieving them, for example, that John Locke (1690) speculated as being a criterion for the non-attribution of personal responsibility and discontinuity of personhood. It is closely associated with contemporary fears of ageing and the supposed link between ageing and dementia. If one cannot remember, in other words, how far can one be thought of as the same, and therefore accountable, person?

The power of life review and reminiscence has become a central element in therapeutic work in later life largely because of this belief in the therapeutic value of memory. However, such opinions were not immediately accepted within gerontology. Erikson's (1963) early remarks about integrating self-experience through the acceptance of 'one's own and only life cycle' and the people who are significant to it took on a radical aspect relative to the dominant perspective of his day. From being seen as a tendency to talk about earlier experience as 'living in the past', as not, in other words, keeping up with the demands of modernist notions of progress and productivity in the present, it has come to characterize the technology for personal integration in later life. Thus, by 1986, Coleman felt able to write that 'An almost totally negative view to talking or thinking about the past has been replaced by a much more positive one' (Coleman 1986: 41).

A number of writers on life review (Butler 1963), autobiographical memory (Salaman 1970; Conway 1990) and group reminiscence behaviour (Coleman 1986) have suggested that the recall of memories from across the lifecourse is a naturally occurring, if not always a welcome, aspect of later life. Dittman-Kholi (1991) has concluded that identities may exist on a different temporal basis in earlier and later adulthood, as older people emphasize continuity with the past more than younger people do, together with a focus on maintenance of identity rather than change and development. This may result in a more realistic sense of self and lowered expectations in later life. In a review of identity management, again by Coleman (1996), it is suggested that 'A satisfactory life story guarantees meaning so long as the link with the past is maintained.' Both the retrieval of memory and a sense of connection between past events and current experience is therefore required for the construction of a meaningful personal narrative. To be convincing, in other words, narratives need to be grounded longitudinally. However, Coleman (1996: 102) goes on to say: 'There is evidence that many old people in our society lack the encouragement they need and the audience to whom to tell their story.' This latter point indicates that spontaneous reminiscence may often be inhibited or driven under cover.

When memory finds a public space, it is often difficult to distinguish between the banal and the profound. Moody (1988) regrets the bowdlerization of life review. He claims that it has come to be used as a means of bolstering cultural myths about the past and the construction of old age that owes more to the psychological needs of the younger listener or collator than the reviewers themselves. It is suggested that the use of reminiscence technology in everything from school projects to residential care has not only become a dominant instituitional means of negotiating intergenerational relationships, but also promotes an underlying message that the present is better than the past and society knows more now than was known then. The power of the past to disturb is thereby simplified and domesticated according to the needs of a dominant and mostly younger age group.

A second, and less utopian, positioning of memory can be found in a growing literature on the relationship between memory and post-traumatic stress in later life (Thompson 1997; Hunt *et al.* 1997). Memories emerging in later life of the holocaust (Hassan 1997), warfare and imprisonment (Robbins 1997) and political violence (Gibson 1997) powerfully express the enduring power of personal traumatic experience of historical events. It would not be possible to understand the behaviour and accompanying psychological pain of these survivors were it not for the legitimizing power of memory and a groundedness in actual historical events.

The association between memory and trauma is, of course, a key component of the psychoanalytic understanding of repression, self-deception and cure. Conway (1990) notes that, according to Freudian interpretation, childhood amnesia arises in response to emotional episodes which an adult would find threatening and disturbing. Such memories are screened by the remembrance of less disturbing events and are thereby hidden from direct retrieval. The original sequence and content of events slides beneath a different set of memories in just the same way as words disguise, yet are linked by association to alternative meanings in the psychoanalytic discourse. Current identities are fashioned less, it would seem, from forgetting than from an inability to forget, plus the unconscious pull exerted by memories that have been repressed. Genuineness, according to this therapeutic discourse, arises through an apprehension of the correct, i.e. the original, ordering of events and their contents. The message in the memory is then understood and individuals are able to assume the role of an active agent, with increased control over their own destiny.

However, Vialdi (1996) has argued that trauma can significantly disrupt notions of the truth and of memory such that it is no longer clear whether memories reflect personally experienced events, the experience of others or fantasy. Through her examination of family secrets, she suggests that adult children may unconsciously act out traumatic parental experiences which have not been verbally conveyed to them for cultural or political reasons. She takes the case of a young woman who repeats behaviours that stem from her mother's past as a political activist who experienced the murder of her relatives, torture and imprisonment. The daughter developed a narrative to explain the gaps and elisions in her family history, which, 'Instead of helping to uncover and dissolve the fantasy, furnishes it with material, and works to obscure the distinction between what belongs to the parent's real experience and what to the child's fantasy' (Vialdi 1996: 36). The adult child's 'memories' become a confusing mixture of actual and imagined events, as 'what returns to haunt the child belongs to somebody else's unconscious'. It no longer becomes possible to distinguish between the reality of the adult child's experience and the residues of that of significant others. The notion of secrets in the family is not new to the psychodynamic approach, and can be found in the work of Pincus and Dare (1978). These authors suggest that unless the chain is broken by a member questioning his or her family's assumptive world, unspoken trauma experienced by earlier generations can inhibit and distort, and lead to the transgenerational repetition of suffering.

Arguments on the contested status of remembering have been extended by exponents of the cultural study of memory (King 1996; Fairhurst 1997). Here there is a marked disregard for original veracity. Instead, a perspective has been adopted that studies the contexts within which memories are produced and the relatedness of content to the context of production. It is not memory itself which is of interest as much as the construction of certain statements and uses of language that denote certain utterances as being labelled as memory. Their interest, however, lies not in how certain memories can be recalled depending upon how the remembering individual judges them to be appropriate, what Gubrium (1993) has called 'communicated lives', as much as in how they arise in language and how that status is conferred. Thus, psychoanalysis is construed by Burman (1996) as being a repository of meanings around narratives of the past and an arbiter of what counts as 'real' memory. Accordingly, traumas are traumatic because they have not been assimilated into a meaningful discourse, rather than the emotional disturbance that surrounded events that occurred and were then repressed.

Memories in this tradition are described in the language of text and surface. They not only become the plaything of whatever narrative is currently being performed in the present, they are bleached of time and personal history. They are words labelled memory, rather than memory represented in words. Memory, in other words, without a notion of the past.

The question of the veracity of recovered memory has been set in sharper contrast by the debate on false memory syndrome (Burman 1996; Crews 1997). Many contemporary psychotherapists might maintain that the strict historical truth of an event is less important to the therapeutic process in the here and now than the patient's belief that it is true. Attention has moved away from the classical psychoanalytic, and archaeological, model of insight through recovery of buried memories, to an understanding of the patient's view of the world. Remembered events can, in other words, become part of a believable narrative and a personal guide for acting in and interpreting the world without being objectively true. What one has to work with, as a therapist, are those guiding principles by which an individual lives his or her life and whether, in the process of therapy, suffering can be reduced and happiness increased.

These assumptions not only obscure the relationship between accurate recollection of the past and the selective aims of the present (Bollas 1989); they have a potentially explosive effect once they travel beyond the psychodynamic session and impact on everyday relationships with others. Examples of the need for a grounding beyond internal logic can be found in the use of memory in the courts, in statutory helping agencies and as they affect other people still living. Here, it makes sense to distinguish between trauma that is covered up and fantasy which is taken for real. In contemporary psychotherapy, the difference between truth or falsity may be incidental. This is not the case in social settings which include points of law and the conduct of others. In the latter case, self-narratives may be recast as untruths unless they are sufficiently rooted in externally verifiable events, and the courtroom is a distinctly un-postmodern environment.

Oral memory of actual historical events can also serve a function of cultural resistance to dominant narratives. This point has been vividly expressed by Corrigan and Leonard (1981), who describe how the memories of older people can inform community and social work understanding of histories of struggle within a locality. These memories are often associated with particular landmarks, or the sites of landmarks that have since disappeared (Dittman-Kholi 1991). Gellhorn (1997: 6) describes, for example, how memories of the British miners' strike struggle for survival against an official attitude of hostility and erasure. 'We all know about history being re-written, but in Wales, history has been turfed over. This place had a mine on every block, it was solid coal: now there's no sign there were ever mines here. It's a most extraordinary example of how history can be erased.' Under such circumstances, memories of the miners' struggle and community spirit may have to rely on communication across generations, a reservoir of collective tactics and strategies that are unlikely to be recorded by official rewritings of the heritage industry. The value of memory is also reflected in studies of migration (Amin and Patel 1998; Blakemore 1998; Comley 1998) where it can have a connective function between generations and sustain 'unofficial' narratives. There is a connection here with the political projects discussed by Andrews (1991) and de Beauvoir (1970) (see Chapter 4) in the suggestion that meaning is given to existence through a continued devotion to social emancipation. Men and women who 'Have been and are still fully involved with living, knowing that even after they die, the fights in which they have been engaged will persist', are, according to this perspective, 'Unlike many others of their age who feel they no longer belong to society, [as] they continue to have a strong purpose in life, a reason for living' (Andrews 1991: 207). Here, the notion of a continued interaction between past and present commitment valorizes memory, in a way that a focus on its relative and insubstantial qualities does not.

Within psychodynamic and social action approaches to identity, here and now relationships resonate with memories and the past. There is an emphasis on continuity and using the past as a guide to understanding the present. Further, memories of experienced events are privileged over remembered dreams, television programmes, novels and other forms of fantasy activity. The relationship between past and present, hidden and apparent, and thus the territory of the masque, is seen as becoming increasingly permeable as it is understood by the active subject. Memory is important within these traditions, but is not necessarily taken to be accurate. Rather, memory is seen as containing truths which are often hidden and whose recovery can lead to an increased realism in everyday life. Memories are valued as a link to the past, and value the experience of longevity. Within the context of postmodernity, however, the value of memory is unclear. It is flattened and used for different purposes, and has no existence outside the coercive force of an unstable present. While memories in mature adulthood can be valued, then, they are not generally so. They emerge, but have no public voice. They exist covertly.

MORTAL FINITUDE

While it can be seen from the above discussion that memory is a contested subject, it can, under certain conditions, represent a form of connectivity. This connectivity looks back, over the shoulder. Its power lies in lessons that can be learned and the undertow of repressed contents. In mature adulthood, the subject must also find a connectivity by looking forwards, which in this lifecourse context means the apprehension of a finite existence. As authors such as Lynch (1997) point out, death is relatively absent from contemporary experience. Most people's contact with it is either abrupt and privatized, or mediated by a bowdlerizing and sensational popular culture. It is not a welcome guest unless it is masked in the conceits of murder mystery or the horror movie. By contrast, the apprehension of death as the ultimate expression of finitude has been the special concern of existential psychotherapists, of whom Yalom (1980) and Frankl (1969) are key.

Within the existential tradition the expression of choice and personal freedom is tempered by the simultaneous experience of limitation. This is not necessarily, as Maquarrie (1973: 148) puts it, 'an observed state of affairs but the inward, existential awareness of one's own being as a fact that is to be accepted.' One simply finds oneself in a limited, factual, corporeal existence and has to come to terms with it as the antidote to fantasies of unlimited possibility. According to this perspective, it would be wrong to understand death as simply a point of termination. It is not relegated to the end of the story, but becomes very much a part of the continuing experience of self. This is in part because, whereas the beginning of the lifecourse can be assigned a definite starting point in the past, it is impossible to tell whether actual existence will extend as far as our future plans or possibly beyond them. Without apprehension that an end-point exists, it would be difficult to gain a sense of personal existence as a whole. The intimation of a limit to life means that things cannot be put off indefinitely. The task that fills the time available to personal existence is couched in terms of achieving authenticity: 'man must decide who he will be, and more than this, each individual must decide the question for himself' (Maquarrie 1973: 161).

Yalom (1980) claims that while death is a core question for existence, it is more often than not one that is avoided both inside and outside the therapeutic situation. He sums this up accordingly: 'Do not patients have quite enough fear and quite enough dread without the therapist reminding them of the grimmest of life's horrors? Why focus on bitter and immutable reality? If the goal of therapy is to instill hope, why evoke hope-defeating death?' (Yalom 1980: 29). It is a view reflected in the responses of counsellors who, while seeing issues of bereavement as closely associated to work with older clients, generally did not focus on the meaning of personal mortality (Woolfe and Biggs 1997).

Against this common-sense position it is argued that life and death are interdependent and exist simultaneously, so that 'death whirs continuously beneath the membrane of life', and also that death is a fundamental source of anxiety which, if left unattended, results in psychopathology. The positive function of an increased awareness of death is that it jolts the individual out of a state of immersion in everyday life. Here, Yalom draws on Heidegger's (1926) distinction between forgetfulness of being and mindfulness of being. It is only in the latter state that one becomes aware of personal authorship and responsibility and can therefore exist authentically. This is because once finitude has been apprehended, the purpose of existence itself can no longer be postponed. Yalom cites a number of examples from his therapeutic practice which illustrate the way in which near-death experiences and group exercises that are aimed to put participants in contact with their own mortality can provoke a re-established connection with meaning and a more fulfilling existence. Classical psychoanalysis, he argues, fails to address these questions because it only looks backwards to past life events for inspiration. It is therefore conceptually unsuited to address questions that project identity into the future. Freud's (1920) conception of Thanatos, or death instinct, in his later work similarly fails to address the existential meaning of finitude because, according to Yalom, he conceived of it primarily as a will to destructiveness in opposition to libidinal wishes towards creation, and not as an encounter with mortality as such.

However, Yalom's approach has been criticized by van Deurzen-Smith (1997: 158) for its reliance on technical fixes and clinical modes of practice which result in 'a list of basic anxieties rather than . . . a framework for living'. It is unclear, then, whether this version of existential psychotherapy allows its subject to address lifecourse problems, which, to paraphrase Jung's (1933a) words, allow one to remain vitally alive by being ready to die with life.

Frankl (1955) places a particular emphasis on finitude as a spur to meaning in life. It is suggested that temporality, the irreversible quality of the lifecourse, 'brings our patients to consciousness of their responsibility'. One cannot undo things that have been done, the consequences of which stay with their author. The nature of this responsibility, responsibility for what exactly, is not always clear in Frankl, other than that it contributes to a search for authentic meaning.

Frankl (1955) agrees with Jung (1933a) that the pervasive malaise of modern existence is its lack of sense of purpose. Thus, a second consequence of finitude appears in its implications for existential projects. If there were no end-point to existence, there would be no particular reason to do anything. Immortals can put things off indefinitely, whereas mortality, and in this case consciousness of mortality, confounds the fantasies of infinite time and a continuous present. Awareness of mortality, it is argued, means that we have to get up and do something. In the doing, and reflection on doing, lies meaning. Van Deurzen-Smith (1997) suggests that three sources of meaning can be found in Frankl's work. These include 'what we give to life', in terms of creative action; 'what we take from the world' through the experience of values, the foremost of which is the opportunity to love; and the stand taken towards 'fate' that can no longer be changed. The notion of 'taking a stand' is seen as key to authenticity, and distinguishes active experience of the world from passive emersion in it. A combination of the power of finitude, the need to take a stand and the experience of temporality leads to Frankl's most famous exhortation: 'the leading maxim of existential analysis might be put thus: live as if you were living for the second time and had acted as wrongly the first time as you are about to act now' (Frankl 1955: 75).

Thus, according to exponents of an existential tradition in psychotherapy, an apprehension of mortality is an essential motor for living. Out of it spring remorse, regret and an urge to learn from mistakes. It is a core ingredient for making sense of the lifecourse and, through an awareness of transience, adds depth and poignancy to the concept of lifecourse itself. To ignore or deny finitude would therefore deny life essential meaning and purpose. Its absence from contemporary Western culture, when wedded to increasing existential potency as the lifecourse progresses, strengthens its candidature as an undercover preoccupation of the mature imagination.

SPIRIT AND TRANSCENDENCE

Intimations of mortality have traditionally been linked to spirituality, and while this has been largely left unaddressed within an existential tradition, it can become a powerful source of connectivity both personally and culturally. Spirituality and ageing have been associated by each of the major world religions, including Christianity (Post 1992), Judaism (Isenberg 1992) and Islamic, Hindu and Buddhist (Thursby 1992) traditions. McFadden (1996) notes that while ageing elicits the sort of existential questions that religion and spirituality seek to answer, and 76 per cent of North Americans declare that religion is very important to them, it has not been a question widely addressed by social gerontology. Indeed, these meaning systems are characterized as losing their power and contributing to an experience of difference and distance between younger and older generations (Marcoen 1994). The displacement of spirituality has become a central goal of modernity, which Moody (1986) links to a 'dual displacement of meaning' in contemporary old age. This consists in the first place of a displacement of leisure and, more notably, contemplation from the rest of the lifecourse into old age and of a simultaneous displacement of death, finitude and judgement from the after-life into later stages of the present life. Accordingly, the burden of life's meaning has been shifted to the end of the lifecourse.

A key component of spirituality concerns a quest for meaning, which McFadden (1996) associates with a 'sense of connection and integration'. He points out that 'elder wisdom, unitative states of consciousness, transcendence and awareness of multiple realities' all indicate the importance of spirituality as part of late-life development. According to this view, religious philosophies have become the road maps that guide the lifecourse in the face of the unknown and intimations of the numinous, as well as performing the social function of stabilizing group behaviour.

Marcoen (1994) has noted that many people who are in late adulthood and old age develop a relationship with transcendent reality which becomes a core element in their 'global personal well-being'. Existential questions that have remained latent in other parts of the lifecourse now arise, and it is claimed that those who have a spiritual outlook on life are more able to prevent negative affects drowning positive feelings, even when the material conditions of life are deteriorating. The power of spirituality lies, it is argued, in the belief that 'A person's spirituality is grounded in the experience of a transcendent relationship to something greater than oneself' (Marcoen 1994: 527).

Elkins *et al.* (1988) have emphasized that spirituality should be seen as a humanistic phenomenon distinguished from religiosity, the participation in the beliefs, rituals and activities of traditional religion. According to this view, spirituality concerns whatever one considers to be the ultimate, and may include ecological concerns and concern for others and for the self. An apprehension of the transcendent 'opens the person to power of myths, metaphors, stories and insights which characterise his or her particular spirituality' (Marcoen 1994: 529). It can thereby become source material around which to cohere a personal narrative. Further,

'The relationship to a transcendent reality guarantees that one keeps feeling loved and precious, even when the effects of the ageing process seem to falsify these self-perceptions. The ageing person who succeeds in living entirely decentred, grounded in something which is greater than himself or herself, will take the unchangeable losses of life as they are, and will courageously live with them, less expansive than before, but concentrated and directed to what really counts in life' (Marcoen 1994: 531).

Ram-Prashad (1995) has surveyed classical Indian philosophical perspectives on ageing and spiritual meaning. Within this tradition, the first three parts of the adult lifecourse gain meaning by being world-oriented, and include studenthood, householding and the stage of the forest dweller. This third stage is almost universally construed as a transitional period, in preparation for the fourth and final stage of renunciation. The final stage of life is thereby devoted to 'world-transcending contemplation'. Renunciation is not thought of as rejection of the sort envisaged by Western notions of disengagement, however. It is not the denial or rejection of life; it is the acceptance of its limited, provisional meaning. The process of ageing can enhance 'Liberation in the sense of freedom from the world of ordinary life and realisation in the sense of the discovery of what the consciousness present in that ordinary life "really" is. The attainment of realisation is tantamount to liberation from a life embedded in this world' (Ram-Prashad 1995: 7).

In other words, an escape from the circularity of material desire and the round of everyday activity characteristic of the first three stages is perceived as being a positive advantage, allowing perception to grow beyond the immediate, the material and the transient. 'Microcosmic meanings', or those that are embedded in everyday existence, do, however, come to be seen as necessary and part of being connected with a wider meaning, if unconsciously so. For example, the role of ritual and moral codes in everyday life is to harmonize these activities with a cosmic order. Awareness of the 'macrocosmic' allows former life phases to be apprehended as being circular and concern with the material as ultimately being meaninglessness beyond itself. This ignites a need to search out those wider meanings through a preparedness to accept one's own life as arbitrary and meaningless and thereby to give up individuality as essentially fleeting and absurd. Ram-Prashad notes that humans apprehend the spiritual at all stages of life, but it is in old age that it becomes relevant. Rather than being caught up in specifics, 'An old individual finds that there are certain broad and general features which mark life but finds too that there are no further reasons for why they have so marked life; they just have' (Ram-Prashad 1995: 29).

The focus on moving beyond material restraints in a search for something greater than the self is similar to that of Sherman and Webb's

(1994) observations on reminiscence. They note that reminiscence reveals life as a process and a spiritual journey for some older people, 'that moves from a possessive attachment to an identification to the physical self, significant others and material belongings, to a view of self as a process, as "being" rather than "having" within and as part of a larger process'(Sherman and Webb 1994: 255).

Thus, it is suggested, through the logic of spirituality, that the attainment of internal consistency is not enough for lifecourse development. Specifically, there is a yearning for some form of connection to a greater reality than can be contained either by immersion in materiality or by an individually cohesive narrative. This search goes beyond the maintenance of continuity and material activity promised by existential psychotherapy. However, it is difficult to find a legitimized space for spirituality within modern or postmodern readings of the lifecourse. Both would force the expression of profound spirituality underground. More often than not modernity has defined itself against spirituality, which is then characterized as superstition or as being unscientific. It has become a casualty of an Enlightenment war against formal religion, which when expressed is rendered pathological. The postmodern 'anything goes' version of identity consumption fails to distinguish between profound and banal experience, rendering spiritual choice profoundly banal. Its materiality and celebration of surface expression leave little space for depth and connectivity to something greater than self; indeed, grander narratives have been treated with considerable suspicion.

FORMS OF CONNECTION AND SOCIABILITY

The spiritual argument that the mature imagination brings with it an awareness and a need for meaning that is greater than the individual is reflected in both mainstream and marginal accounts of lifecourse development. It is possible to read Eriksonian generativity in this light. Erikson (1963) and Kotre (1984) have both interpreted generativity as an interest in establishing and guiding the next generation, the failure of which leads to stagnation. This view links generative life tasks to immortality, as children and grandchildren come to be seen as an extension of the self and thus as a source of influence and control over the termination of the material self. Alexander *et al.* (1992: 425) critically describe this process as 'A way of infusing the self into the other with the hope that it will live on forever.' It is a symbolic act, though not necessarily a conscious one aimed at creating an enduring and infinite self through an investment in the other. They argue, however, that there is no altruism present, but a culturally specific notion of self-perpetuation.

Woolger's (1987) accounts of the discovery of past lives through psychotherapy can be seen as another, though distinctly un-modern, attempt to extend the self beyond a single lifecourse. It is argued that previous lives leave physical and psychological traces in current existence which need to be discovered if a patient is to obtain relief. Here, we have the trauma model extended to spiritual cleansing, which, by extension, will lead to happier future lives and thereby solve the problem of finitude.

The original psychoanalytic explanation of trauma and repression relied heavily on sexuality. This is rarely considered as a source of contemporary psychological disturbance (Frosh 1991; Zaretsky 1997), and is seen as content that is itself contextually dependent on conditions at the time of Freud's original writings. It is, however, possible that the overt expression of sexuality continues to be a problem for many older adults. This is not as much due to the unacceptable nature of such thoughts to the individual themselves, however, as to a contemporary culture that perceives later life as a period of asexuality (Greer 1991). Aitman (personal communication), for example, when asked to write a series of pamphlets on psychological issues in later life, had proposals for copy on sexuality in old age rejected as too contentious. At least one training video on intimacy in residential care construes male sexuality as primarily a nuisance to staff and other residents (Samdersen 1994). Some of the most cutting ageist stereotypes and popular catch phrases (mutton dressed as lamb, dirty old man, cradle-snatcher) have been reserved for sexuality and age. Pointon (1997: 7), in a review of sexuality and later life, suggests that 'Negative attitudes surrounding older people and sexuality can result in the mistaken belief among older people themselves that sex stops at sixty.' Legitimized sexual activity, it appears, ends with that great modern lifecourse divider, retirement. This is, of course, a modern myth debunked by a series of studies (Masters and Johnson 1970; Brecher 1993; Kaye 1993) which indicate that sexual activity and desire persist into deep old age. It is a myth, however, that can have serious consequences not just for the expression of sexuality in general, but is particularly threatening when it restricts access to services established to care primarily for the young, such as AIDS (Marshall 1997). The implication for surface and hidden aspects of identity is that sexuality is required to exist surreptitiously beneath an asexual masquerade. It is a form of connection which is often unrecognized, and in the public arena is subject to powerful sources of informal control.

It will be recalled that within the tradition of analytical psychology, ageing, and most notably adult psychological maturation, is construed through the concept of increasing individuation. It is possible to interpret individuation as being dominated by the quest for the internal logic of the personal psyche; a reading of the process through the application of the techniques of active imagination, as attempted by Weaver (1973) and Chodorow (1997), positively encourages such a view. This is, however, only a partial exploration of the process as a whole. Samuels *et al.* (1986) suggest a social dimension to this process that might otherwise be over-looked. As individuation progresses, they argue, 'The person becomes conscious in what respects he or she is both a unique human being and, at the same time, no more than a common man or woman' (Samuels *et al.* 1986: 76). So while, as Jung points out in *Psychological Types* (1921), the goal of the process is the development of the individual personality, it presupposes that this includes and is grounded in collective relation-ships. The opposition to social conformity found in Jung's mistrust of the persona should not, in other words, preclude social connection as an ultimate psychological goal. It is not a shutting out of the world, but a gathering in around the seat of personal consciousness, and in this sense is a psychological correlate of de Beauvoir's (1970) social action.

There are a number of ways in which increased individuation can lead to increased sociability. According to Samuels (1985), for example, the perception of others does not simply include internally generated arche-types; psychological blueprints that prefigure an understanding of the social world. These are filled out, made into a fuller picture, by percep-tions of others as they are experienced in direct relationships with the active subject. Others are also, over time, increasingly perceived as separ-ate persons in their own right. Indeed, the increased self-acceptance that individuation describes leads to a return of psychological projections and thus to a perception of others that is less cluttered by personal prejudice. An increasing sense of dialogue between inner and outer realities affects both internal psychological processes and perceptions of the social world. Weaver (1973) points out that it is increasingly possible to distinguish between the internalized social world and one's own thoughts and moods. An internal dialogue can then take place between these images that have been adopted as social archetypes and a person's own sense of self. By using the metaphors of analytic psychology, one can make sense of a maturational process that includes increasing distinction between aspects of experience, so that an individual is not swamped by emotions and prejudices, and achieves an increased ability to connect with others as persons and groupings in their own right.

IMPLICATIONS: FROM REFLEXIVITY TO REFLECTIVITY

This review of some of the candidates for the essentially unexpressed, the hidden yet psychologically alive, logics of the mature psyche has identified memory of the past, apprehension of the future and connectiv-ity with the social as contested sources of personal continuity. It suggests that one's story is not entirely one's own and that in order to develop a mature imagination links need to be made to something greater than the self. This process is redolent with uncertainty, insofar as openness to wider association requires a readiness to accept things beyond personal control. Maturity may thus be exhibited in an ability to tolerate such forms of indeterminacy.

An increased permeability is also suggested between depth and surface. In the language of the masque, this would indicate that personae and the performance of masquerade include elements of the hidden in their tentative journey to connect with authentic sites for expression. An example of permeability also exists in the proposed connection of past, present and future; not, however, in the service of immediate impression management as much as in an attempt at moulding cohesion and continuity into a sense of grounded personal coherence. Flexibility of surface components of identity thus comes to complement the elusive, yet potent, logic of deeper psychological layering.

While psychoanalysis constitutes a now longstanding method, or technology, for getting beyond appearances, it is flawed in terms of the mature imagination insofar as the significance of memory and future behaviours is reduced to repetition of past and most notably childhood experience. As an essentially modern project, the object of mainstream psychoanalysis is to escape the past rather than live with it. However, in ceasing to allow memory to have a logic of its own, postmodern criticism commits an equally brutal form of closure. In the lifecourse manifestation of midlifestyle, for example, the personal past and future are subject to an exercise of almost surgical removal and forgetting. The result is a continuous recycling of identity that is decreasingly grounded in a reality outside itself.

There are, according to the current view, no neat conclusions and no neat answers to what is behind the mask. The question demands careful handling rather than iconoclastic deconstruction and if identities are synthetically created, questions must be asked about why and how they work. There may be considerable authenticity in the way people think about and experience their constructed identities even if they are not on grounds of their own choosing. A focus on permeability would redirect attention to the connection of internal logic and the intersubjectively real. They are interdependent and symbiotic in character. There is an internal logic to the intersubjective and an internal logic to deeper psychological processes, which sometimes finds expression when the two logics resonate with a particularly hospitable social space. If this is not the case, they run along parallel paths and can become increasingly separate.

If a consideration of the relationship between depth and surface suggested here requires the recognition of the permeability of mature identities, then there is also a change in emphasis from the reflexivity of contemporary social identity to a consideration of the role of reflectivity. Reflectivity includes the notion of a longitudinal component to the construction of the self in a way that reflexivity does not. Indeed reflexivity, as a process intimately related to the recycling of identities in the present, is fundamentally compromised in this respect. Reflection, and the self-conscious creation of spaces for reflection, is inimicable to the onward rush of immediate social experience. It allows the active subject to stand back from the flow and to see the pattern in events rather than being swept along by them. It demands the ability to tolerate disruption of the continuous procession. In this sense, reflectivity rescues a belief that personal histories can inform the present, or at least indicate the dangers implicit in certain actions and positions. The past can, in other words, be used to interpret possible futures, and insofar as ageing constitutes a connection to past experience and has come to occupy a similar space in the popular imagination, the fortunes of the two processes are closely tied together.

The rescuing of reflection allows here and now relationships to resonate with the memories and aspirations of participants, a process that assumes that memories and sequences of memory largely retain their original meanings but also merge with immediate experience. The apprehension of continuity acts as a guide and is made available through reflection. It is a reality that, while being personal, is privileged over fragments arising from dreams, television, novels and the notion that selves can be reinvented through the neo-psychotic processes of internal logic alone.

7

Social spaces and mature identity

THE HIDDEN, THE SURFACE AND SOCIAL SPACE

An enduring theme within this book is that the mature imagination has, throughout different historical periods and when seen through different social and philosophical lenses, encountered different possibilities for expression. The relationship between ageing and the social spaces available to the performance of identity is, however, a dynamic one. Attempts to fix notions of adult ageing interact reflexively with the identities that are their object, such that both are modified over time. Different ideas of and policies towards ageing contribute to the creation of a social space, a sort of arena in which performances of identity achieve public recognition and, in a Foucauldian (1977) sense, are legitimized.

In the case of the psychodynamic tradition, it would appear that classical psychoanalysts first rejected serious consideration of an intrinsic subjectivity of adulthood and with it the possibility of fruitful work with mature adults. There then followed a period marked by revision, in which the reach of the psychodynamic project was extended to include groups, such as older people, who had previously occupied only its margins. In recent years, classical psychoanalysis has itself all but been rejected as an inappropriate and restrictive paradigm for such work. It has given way to more flexible and age-sensitized forms of therapy.

Simply using the phrase, 'possibilities for expression', however, assumes a certain type of relationship between personal identity and social context. This is because it is implicitly accepted that there is some core seat of consciousness, of selfhood, from which the social world can be apprehended and reflected upon. This core sense of self is itself a meeting point of the explicitly known and the tacitly, intuitively or unconsciously felt. The degree to which tacit, or hidden, aspects of this self can find expression in outer as well as inner experience would depend on the particular contexts that are available to the performance of identity. The degree of direct expression that takes place, the inflection or nuance given to self-expression and in some cases the possibility of expression at all are intimately related to the quality of the social spaces that emerge. It is this relationship between those self-attributes that have become core and the social spaces that already exist or can be created which determines whether a performed identity is experienced as genuine or not.

The determination of the genuine is contested within contemporary literature on identity. Within the psychodynamic tradition, pride of place is given to the core, the ontological seat of identity, the inner life of the person. It is assumed that there are certain internal priorities, which have variously been labelled drives, desires or potentials, that take precedence when one is theorizing the relationship between self and social space. In other words, the psychodynamic perspective consists of looking out from the inside. Moral authority is given to the emerging self, struggling against the circumstances in which it finds itself. The approach does, however, tend to emphasize the origins of identity and underplay the social construction of spaces in which it is performed. Other theoretical positions, which might include symbolic interactionism and Goffmanesque dramaturgical approaches, appear to start from the opposite pole. Privilege is given to the external social environment in determining genuineness. Self-expression appears to subsist on a terrain of discourses which determine the degree of successful fit between the inner and the outer. Self-expression becomes the deployment of strategies that function to assimilate the quirky and irrational into a socially situated self. However, this form of theorizing is marked by a failure to distinguish substantially between social conformity and genuine self-expression. A postmodern solution to this problem can be seen in the multiplication of spaces for the performance of identity and the unpeeling of meanings from their original significance. So, rather than the argument being that mature adulthood is achieved through an increased awareness of previously unexpressed parts of the self or an adoption of predefined social stereotypes, it is argued that memory, embodiment and locality can be consumed to suit whatever identity statement suits immediate circumstances. The limits to consumption, however, are still externally defined and the question of personal agency and its attendant concerns of responsibility and free will, twin contributors to what is commonly understood by genuine self-expression, has been insubstantially sketched out.

The current argument explores the relationship between the personal and the social in terms of the balance that can be achieved between what is hidden and what can be expressed. How far, in other words, can personal experience connect with something bigger than itself? What is the role of social reality, which is itself bigger than the individual and creates a space for mature identity, in the likelihood that this will happen? What opportunities arise to reflect upon this process and connect it to an understanding of the past and the future? As adult identity develops, it appears that the priorities of earlier adulthood mutate into a different and mature form. Yet, even as this happens, social spaces are contested by alternative and often antagonistic agendas and the particular priorities of later life are driven underground by those of other age groups. The expression of this age-based antagonism is multilayered and can occur in debates over social expenditure (Minkler and Robertson 1991), the responses of users and workers in social and health services (Hughes 1995), the privileging of childhood experience in theory (Biggs 1998) and the adoption of midlifestyles (Featherstone and Hepworth 1990).

At an individual level, tension might occur between a desire for personal continuity and the presentation of a cohesive narrative in the mature adult's immediate situation. Possibilities of engaging in a relatively unselfconscious performance of identity would be reduced where that identity jarred with an age-structured commonsense reality. Under such circumstances, the deployment of social masking also takes on a an age-specified meaning which is expressed in a particular layering of the adult psyche. Some things have to be hidden and some things can be expressed. Some things become tacit in social situations and some explicit. This, it has been suggested, can result in parallel forms of logic which contain their own forms of intrinsic consistency. By degrees, such layering results in an intersubjectively determined presentation of identity which might bear little resemblance to the dynamic of the personal, inner world.

This understanding of the mature imagination presents the relationship between inner and outer logics of self-identity in a new way, posing the question of social space in terms of the likelihood of genuine self-expression becoming possible. Likelihood, as has been touched on in Chapter 4, concerns the balance between the protective and the connective qualities of a social mask. The performance of masquerade, in other words, forms links between the external social world and the internal desires of the performer, while at the same time shielding the inner life from external threat and assault. Social masking and its performance through masquerade become critical in the management of the boundary between self and other, and the permeability of that boundary reflects the possibilities latent in any one social space available for identity performance. When the social environment is hostile, the protective function is emphasized and the boundary becomes fixed and rigid. If a sympathetic social space arises, the connective function becomes ascendant and the boundary becomes more permeable. Another way of putting this is that under hospitable circumstances the inner and outer logics of mature identity are able to run together and thereby become amenable to simultaneous and harmonious expression. Within the language of hidden and surface, this is about as close as one gets to a definition of a genuine connection between personal and social realities.

This line of thought leads to consideration of the kinds of social spaces that are available for the development of a mature imagination, the influences on the shapes that they take and the types of performance that can be contained within them. In preceding chapters, the term 'masque' has been used rather loosely to span both the adoption of a particular persona and the performance of masquerade, a sort of semantic arena in which these two meanings can be contained. It has, in other words, been used to mark out the circumference of any one mature identity. This notion of masque is closely related to social space as currently conceived. Masque interacts with social space, rather like the way in which social masking can form a bridge between the personal and the social worlds. Whereas masque would tend to reflect longitudinal differences in the flexibility and content of an ageing identity, spaces refer to different deployments, different permeabilities and different degrees of indeterminacy, security and autonomy in the here and now.

The social space contributes to the shaping of the masque, but is often, and most typically, pre-existent in social terms. It is, more often than not, already intersubjectively formed, agreed upon by other social actors and concrete in terms of policy, the distribution of material resources such as income or the built environment and the social distribution of power. The masque, as a dynamic structuring of identity, is held in the force field of these contingent, but prefiguring, factors. The stronger the forces, the more fixed the relations that take shape. Further, forces may reconfigure, leading to the creation of different spaces and requiring the creation of a different legitimizing masque. Changes in social policy, professional attitudes, lifestyles and self-definitions of ageing all contribute to the shape of age as a social space and the performances that can emerge within it.

In terms of likelihood, this analysis provokes certain questions about what is hidden and what is expressed, which voices can be heard and which voice has to be adopted to be heard. The sort of information that is being communicated, how genuine it is and whether it can be built on as a basis for enduring relationships and future plans have implications for performed identity. They also affect the quality of communication between professional workers and service users and information collected through mechanisms such as quality assurance and partnership arrangements in service systems. Attention is focused on the durability of the spaces that are formed, whether they can be relied upon, whether there is a space for a mature imagination and if so what sort of space, the degree to which it allows the possibility of a synthesis of the masque and the hidden.

THE PSYCHODYNAMIC AND THE SOCIAL

In psychodynamic thinking, the idea that certain spaces can in some way hold particular thoughts and feelings has become key to understanding the relationship between personal and social worlds. It also follows the expansion of psychodynamic ideas from work with individuals, through the development of therapy groups and towards an explanation of organizational and wider social behaviour.

Psychodynamic theory and practice have been dedicated to the creation of containing spaces which act as a laboratory for self-conscious reflection. The concept of a containing space includes the notion that previously unconscious thoughts and emotions can be experienced if a suitably safe place is created, usually by the therapist. This safe place then acts as a container that protects these experiences from external threats to the psyche and allows them to be understood more easily.

If the psychoanalytic session is a self-consciously artificial yet specialized space for examining one-to-one interactions, then the concept of containing space opens the possibility that other reflective and specifically social environments also exist.

Attempts to expand on this relationship between the personal and the social have led writers (Rioch 1970; Stokes 1994; Symington and Symington 1996) to draw heavily on the now seminal work of Wilfred Bion (1961). Bion believed that group behaviour involved three sets of conflict: that which occurs within the individual, that between the individual and the group and that between the explicit task of the group and its basic assumptions. These thoughts developed while Bion worked within the British armed forces during the Second World War, and first appeared in a series of essays presented to the Tavistock Clinic between 1948 and 1951. He described a group as being 'An aggregate of individuals all in the same state of regression' (Bion 1961: 142).

Bion was, in other words, cautious as to the status of feelings that emerge in group contexts. He did not claim that somehow groups create their own cultures and climates, but rather that this 'same state of regression' gave rise to the fantasy that 'the group' as an autonomous entity existed over and above the experiences of individual members. In this sense he was both respecting the tenet of the psychoanalytic tradition that the individual was to be the principle focus of study and going on to examine new and, for the time, unfamiliar territory. The notion that a group might itself have feelings that hold sway over its members was seen as a mistaken belief that allowed participants to lose their individual distinctiveness and sense of personal responsibility. To explain social phenomena, Bion proposed that when people meet in a group, there are in fact two groups going on.

First, there is the 'work group'. This concerns activities that are used to address the formal task of the group, the reason why it is meeting, and includes attempts to engage with explicit problem-solving. Thus, in a therapy group, for example, 'It can always be seen that some mental activity is directed to the solution of the problems for which the individuals seek help' (Bion 1961: 144). Second, there is activity that is not concerned with this principal function. Individuals hold 'basic assumptions' about what they consciously or unconsciously desire the group to be about, and these assumptions often impede or actively disrupt work group functioning. Stokes (1994) has suggested that group meetings in which the passing of time seems not to be recognized, external realities are ignored or denied, where there is an absence of any real progress and where questioning attitudes are perceived to be foolish, mad or heretical are probably under the sway of basic assumptions of some sort. Bion himself proposed that groups under the influence of basic assumption thinking characteristically take three different forms: dependency, fight–flight and pairing. Dependency is characterized as avoiding development through participants being 'United in the belief that if they sit there long enough, the wise leader will come forth with a magic cure'; fight–flight includes the assumption that the group has 'met to preserve itself and that this can be done only by fighting someone or something or by running away'; in pairing it is assumed that the group has 'met for the purposes of reproduction, to bring forth a saviour' (Bion 1961: 24). In each case the basic assumption, which is often tacit, rather than being an explicit strategy, avoids engagement with the explicit work task of the group.

In terms of the relationship between the personal and the collective, Bion's work marks an important recognition that group, as well as individual, behaviours reflect unconscious psychological processes. Psychodynamic approaches can be used not simply to diagnose society as if it were one big patient or pathology, as was the case with Freud's (1930) *Civilization and Its Discontents*, but as a way of understanding the processes of group behaviour. Bion's insights have been expanded by other psychoanalytically trained workers, such as Jaques (1955) and Menzies (1970). Both of these writers attempted to use psychodynamic thinking to examine the workings of organizations, rather than small groups. Jaques (1955) proposed that social systems – including institutions, such as businesses, hospitals or ships at sea – acted as a defence against forms of persecutory and depressive anxiety. They therefore protected their members from negative feelings that might overwhelm the performance of their original task, while also becoming something of a hothouse for various forms of personally threatening projections if these processes are not recognized. The occupants of certain roles, most notably ones centred on issues of leadership, will come to attract negative transference and bad impulses, projected by other members of a social system on to these key figures. Those figures then come to contain these attributes for the rest of the organization, allowing it to continue working, if in a rather dysfunctional manner.

Menzies (1970), following a study of nursing within a 'general teaching hospital in London', suggested that social systems in hospitals and other institutions can act as defences against the anxiety of those who work within them. Because work in hospital settings involves a large number of potentially distressing events, such as intimate bodily contact and functions, the anxieties of patients' relatives, envious feelings towards the cared for and the hopes and fears engendered by treatment itself, Menzies argued that means of defending oneself against their impact have become part of the institutional culture. The logic of this way of thinking about the relationship between the social and the personal follows the route that certain social experiences evoke primitive (in the sense of neonatal) emotions and fears, people seek to avoid such situations and over time these characteristic habits of avoidance take institutional forms. Thus, according to this view, 'the characteristic feature of the social defence system . . . is its orientation to helping the individual avoid the experience of anxiety, guilt, doubt and uncertainty (Menzies 1970: 24). Paradoxically, the evolution of institutional defences, such as the wearing of uniforms, stereotyped professional behaviour, frequent changes of shift and workplace, which work to distance nurses from emotional contact with their patients, can mean that underlying anxieties are not confronted and the system maintains a certain level of dysfunction.

Menzies's monograph has since become key to understanding the shaping of social systems within the psychodynamic tradition. It has allowed a link to be made between predominantly work-related cultures and psychological processes, has allowed a space for the irrational in otherwise rationalistic conceptions of organization and has facilitated an understanding of what Lawrence (1995) has called the 'rational madness' of work communities. Woodhouse and Pengelly (1991) draw extensively on it in their study on interprofessional collaboration, Obholzer and Roberts (1994) have studied individual and organizational stress in the human services and Tudor and Tudor (1995) have extended an emphasis on containing anxiety to the study of social services. Social systems are conceived as both containing and constituting defences against forms of anxiety that would otherwise fragment the individual psyche and prevent an agency from addressing its core task.

In the study of human services, it has been recognized that the internal dynamic of any one organization is also affected by common characteristics of the client group being served and the professional groupings working within it. Stokes (1994), for example, has linked Bion's basic assumptions to the cultures of different helping professions. He suggests that dependency is most often associated with nursing and health professionals, fight and flight with social work and pairing with quasi-psychotherapeutic cultures. Mattinson and Sinclair (1979) have expanded on the relationship between agency culture and client group. It is suggested that processes similar to transference and countertransference have led to the preoccupations of any one group of people with similar problems – such as marital problems, instances of child abuse or forms of mental illness or incapacity – being acted out within the organization itself. Forms of rivalry, the avoidance of certain difficult problems or the adoption of characteristic styles and nuances come to mark out the culture of agencies in a characteristic way that reflects the problems experienced by their chosen patients or clients. This process has been labelled 'mirroring', and it is suggested that key conflicts and patterns are mirrored in the agencies' own working practices that arise, yet are not recognized as arising, from the nature of their work.

These developments within the psychodynamic tradition have linked the social and the personal in a particular way. Large social systems provoke and simultaneously contain the acting out of very basic anxieties and desires that are seen as being rooted in individual psychological experience. It thus has a tendency to be linear in its attribution of causality, insofar as institutional defences, while appearing to be social and having a life of their own, are in the final analysis reduced to individual psychological processes. This, most notably in the work of Menzies (1970), is also reduced to the re-enactment of infantile defences against anxiety.

This view has been criticized by Jaques (1995: 343), who now claims that, rather than individuals 'concocting' organizations as a means of collusive defence, 'it is badly organised social systems that arouse psychotic anxieties and lead to their disturbing acting out and expression in working relationships.' In other words, it is not that the containing space of social organization is created to deal with unacceptable fear and desire, but that the spaces created in society are insufficiently caring or robust to allow the development of non-pathological coping.

In a similar vein, Cooper (1996) has criticized the traditional psychodynamic perspective on organizations as being unduly functionalist, such that individuals are seen to be psychologically well insofar as they fit the organizational structure that they find themselves in. This view echoes Zaretsky's (1997) critique that psychoanalysis was once a radical, but is now a conservative, force, and has found its niche in helping people to cope with the stresses on identity induced by late capitalism.

An understanding of the dynamics of social systems has also led, in the work of Miller and Rice (1967) and of Lawrence (1979, 1995) to a view which, while recognizing the dynamic and often unconscious components of social and organizational behaviour, does not link them to childhood or exclusively individual experience. Miller and Rice (1967) and their co-workers (Roberts 1994a) have developed the heuristic concept of a primary task for social systems. This is most easily apprehended by asking: what is it that a helping agency is set up to do, what is its stated purpose? Once a primary task has been identified, it allows the student of organizations to 'Explore the ordering of multiple activities . . . to construct and compare different organisational models of an enterprise' (Miller and Rice 1967: 62).

Lawrence (1977) has argued that it is possible for different people in an organization to pursue different primary tasks as they understand them, which helps us to understand discrepancies between what organizational policy says is happening and what appears to be happening at any one time. There are clearly family resemblances here with Bion's distinction between work and basic assumption thinking, in the sense that priority is, somewhat uncritically, given to formal tasks that are deemed to progress the functioning of an institution. Roberts attempts to clarify the role of primary task by writing that 'The primary task relates to survival in relation to the demands of the external environment, while basic assumption activity is driven by the demands of the internal environment and anxieties about psychological survival . . . where there are problems with the definition of the primary task, there are likely to be problems with boundaries, so that instead of facilitating task performance, they serve defensive functions' (Roberts 1994a: 31, 35).

She addresses the relationship between basic assumptions and primary tasks, and further engages with external social processes, but does not clearly distinguish between primary task and the work group. While there may be misunderstandings over the nature of the task, it appears that both primary task and work configure the nature of that task as, at root, both unitary and unproblematic. The value of the primary task is, according to Lawrence (1979: 10), that it disperses group mythology and an immersion in immediate experience. 'An individual who is in touch with, or holds inside himself, a conception of primary task will be very much involved in the here and now, but will be trying to relate it realistically to the past and the future.' Thus, while the conception of a primary task is problematic in the sense of being unidirectional, it includes an attempt to join the temporal logic of past and future to the logic of the immediate social situation.

Each of the authors above has been active in developing an open systems approach to examining group processes, rather like the way in which the psychotherapy session is used as a tool to put intrapsychic functioning into sharper focus than in everyday life. Here, large groups of participants examine the influence of systems dynamics in what have come to be called group relations conferences. Lawrence (1979: 11) has suggested that such groups make it possible to 'Hear, with the "third ear", what is taking place in the wider society. The large group is a frame for catching what is unconsciously taking place in society at large even though that is not the stated preoccupation nor is life in society the topic of discussion.' Large groups and organizations, in other words, can act as a sort of psychic net, catching wider social phenomena, which then influence conduct within them. In studying group culture one is also studying these tacit influences from wider social processes. Lawrence (1995) has gone on to examine what he calls 'social dreaming': that is, the dreams held in common by members of the same agency, business or professional group. Participants meet and discuss their dreams from the night before; commonalities are noted and are seen to contribute to an understanding of otherwise unconscious social processes. According to Lawrence, these meetings become a container for thoughts that cannot be received elsewhere.

Meanwhile, Khaleelee and Miller (1985) have indicated that groups can be used as 'listening posts' to render societal phenomena an intelligible field of study. Listening posts consist of groups of people who meet to create a reflective space that allows them to distinguish between ephemeral and enduring social influences on their behaviour from wider group cultures. Greater insight would thus be gained about tacit social assumptions as well as overt cultural content. This method was originally developed so that members of organizations could listen in to assumptive realities or the psychological climate of their workplace, but has now been extended by Dartington (personal communication, 1997) and others, such as Palmer (personal communication, 1998), to examine the unconscious influence of societal rather than organizational culture. It is as if, to paraphrase Dartington, it is no longer possible to think of one's mood as being exclusive and personal. Any conversation must now imply or depict a wider context, the speaker's society, which contains tacit or unconscious influences as well as conscious ones and can be named through reflection and interpretation.

In the long journey from the workings of the individual mind to the power of tacit social processes, workers in the psychodynamic tradition have attempted to construct an understanding of the internal dynamics of social spaces and, on occasion, the relationship between what goes on within these spaces, such as groups, agencies, organizations and institutions, and wider-ranging societal processes. These processes are not necessarily considered to be overt cultural phenomena; instead, attention has been focused on an emerging dynamic between events and the tacit social assumptions that they might represent.

It appears from this analysis that the concept of containing space can be used to describe socially occurring spaces, which sometimes cohere around existing institutions and sometimes exist relatively autonomously in the field of social experience, which would include the concept of ageing itself. While apprehension of these spaces, which have psychosocial as well as material presence, is often only tacit in everyday life, opportunities for reflective containment can also make them explicit and available for critical analysis.

AGEING AND THE PSYCHODYNAMIC APPROACH TO SOCIAL SYSTEMS

While listening posts and social dreaming have not, to the author's knowledge, been used specifically with older adults, there are some studies that indicate a particular social dynamic between workers and older people. Dartington (1986) has studied relations between carers for mentally infirm elders and multidisciplinary teams, concluding that 'professionals can bring with them inappropriate attitudes, seeing relatives as a resource to be trained to do better and carry on for longer, rather than people under stress with needs of their own' (Dartington 1986: 37). Sayers (1994) undertook in-depth interviews with those looking after a dementing spouse at home. She examined the defences used by workers and carers looking after persons who are 'emotionally cut off, regressed, anxious, disinhibited or depressed'. These psychological states affect what carers seek from and can use by way of professional support. Findings did not show expected differences between men and women; instead, coping was associated with carers who could attune 'themselves to their partner's state of mind without fear of succumbing to it' (Sayers 1994: 133). In other cases there was a tendency to reproduce the cut-offness experienced by the carer in relations with the dementing elder, such that partners were left in a state of 'incommunicado' and, it is suggested, this dynamic is also present in service systems. Sayers draws on Biggs's (1991) critique of case management as being an insufficiently sensitive method of care when dealing with the emotional dynamic of such situations. She is concerned that managerialist techniques of care fail to provide reflective spaces in which workers and carers alike can examine the psychological impact of their relationships.

The tendency for the needs and indeed presence of older adults in social systems of care to be overlooked is an enduring observation in this literature which may not be completely explained by the presence of dementia. Itzin (1986) and Biggs (1990b) have observed the difficulties that members of age-awareness groups can have in putting themselves in the place of older adults, and the resistance often experienced to work with older adults. Factors such as an irrational fear of personal ageing, an absence and avoidance of disconfirming experiences and the unacceptability of characteristics associated with the second half of life have been suggested (Biggs 1989) as contributing to a general situation in which younger adults simply ignore elders' thoughts, feelings and aspirations. The experience of ageing is thus constituted as an experience of absence.

Miller (1993) and Roberts (1994b) have both consulted to institutions in which older people lived. They report social systems as prone to splitting and fragmentation. In each case, there was a marked absence of communication between different parts of the service system and considerable antagonism between groups of staff who considered themselves to be working with the 'good' patients or with the 'bad' ones. There is a remarkable similarity between these two reports in that it appeared that care for patients who were perceived as being 'incurable' contradicted the ethos of health care systems. The primary task of cure and its attendant reward of optimism were perceived to be lacking in work with some older patients. 'Good' patients were placed on rehabilitation programmes and thereby left the system. 'Bad' ones were left on back wards and perceived as blockages in the system, and their staff considered themselves forgotten and unappreciated. Roberts (1994b) attempted to negotiate a more inclusive primary task, whereas Miller (1993) began to explore both sides of the boundary between the institution and community. Unfortunately, both efforts at consultation were drawn to a premature close. Biggs (1993b) similarly observed a fragmentation of community outreach services for older patients and their carers, such that carers were the only participants in a multidisciplinary consultation who contained the need for continuity of care and held valuable information about the gaps in service provision. An attempt was made to assert the primacy of the active patient as a focus for shared professional tasks. However, the consultation was again ended somewhat prematurely owing to wider service reorganizations.

Perhaps the most enduring and poignant record of consultation to services for vulnerable older adults can be found in the work of Terry (1997, 1998). Terry undertook direct counselling with older patients and worked with management and staff in a consultative capacity over a number of years. As is accepted practice within this tradition, he closely observed his own emotional responses to the environments in which he worked as an aid to understanding the transference and countertransference provoked by such a culture. He notes: 'The anguish of trying to continue an "ordinary" life on these long stay wards when so much has gone and when faced with so many endings and goodbyes; it is so painful that many prefer to withdraw into passivity and mutism' (Terry 1997: 112) .

Staff 'Often split off and denied a capacity to think about their patient's feelings in order to protect themselves from the distress of empathising with their patient's emotional pain' (Terry 1997: 116). The capacity to think about feelings and contain thoughts of despair became located in Terry. They were left with him so that others could 'get on' with institutional life. He increasingly fell prey to intimations of helplessness, hypochondria and a sense of being ignored, as reflections of the emotions experienced by the patients themselves. Through a series of staff support groups, attempts were made to create containers in which these feelings could be discussed with varying degrees of success. However, there are indications in the text that at least part of the reaction to this intervention was to engage in the provision of 'an exciting environment in which there would be no space for sad feelings' (Terry 1998: 120).

This solution is reminiscent of Miller and Gwynne's (1972) study of residential institutions for physically handicapped adults. Two sorts of regimes were observed. The first, referred to as warehousing, was described by authors as a 'social death sentence', in which clients were maintained predominantly through bodily care until physical death actually occurred. The second, referred to as a humanitarian or 'horticultural' culture, encouraged engagement in challenging activity. However, staff often set goals which took little account of clients' physical requirements and capacities, thus creating situations of relative failure. In both cases a rigid distinction between 'normal' and 'abnormal' adulthood was maintained, which defended staff against putting themselves in the position of the other.

Terry (1998) continued to consult staff through a period in which services were privatized. He interpreted privatization as a means through which wider health care systems reproduce the same tendency to deny the potentially disturbing presence of older patients. This presence was considered incompatible with the primary task of hope and cure so central to helping agencies, such that when the opportunity arose patients were evacuated from the system altogether.

The reports noted above bear witness to the heuristic power of the concept of primary task and of looking at the dynamic relationship between persons and systems. However, even within these reports, there is a tendency to hear the voices of younger professionals and a migration away from older adults. Each of the interventions, for example, ended up working principally with staff groups. From a psychodynamic perspective, one is provoked to ask where the containing space for older and particularly vulnerable older adults might be. It is becoming clear that in connecting the social and the psychodynamic, these workers are discovering a complex web of age-segregation, unthought consequences and institutional defences which both contribute to and ask questions of social policy as creating social space.

MATURE IDENTITY AND THE WELFARE STATE

Within the conceptual framework of containing environments, social policy can be construed as an attempt to shape the space in which ideas are articulated, self-expression takes place and relationships are formed around certain legitimised topics. The welfare state, which for these purposes includes both health and social care, can be seen as a place in which society attempts to achieve some form of closure around questions of vulnerability and incapacity. Both are related to the fears, as well as the realities, of adult ageing and contribute to any reconfiguration of ageing, its expression and the social spaces in which it might be recognized.

A number of writers, most notably Phillipson (1982, 1998) in the UK, Estes (1979; Estes *et al.* 1993) and Minkler (1996) in the USA and Kondratowitz (1998) in Germany, have argued that the social space created for ageing, and most particularly ageing after retirement, is closely related to the shape and character of the welfare state. From this perspective, social policy has two functions. First, it enables responses to be made by nominated agencies, in the UK local authority social service departments. In other words, it discriminates between key institutions, such as health, welfare and criminal justice, and gives permission for certain forms of action to take place. These responses will be shaped by the culture and allocations of resources that already exist, what these institutions see as their legitimate domain and expertise. Second, social policy will tend to shape social problems in the public mind. It will reinforce certain beliefs about an issue and underplay others; it will create an environment within which certain legitimate claims and voices can be heard.

Social and historical trends in social policy have assumed a massive break in personal identity and its connection to wider society, with chronological age as the trigger. Under the post-war welfare consensus, the status of adult ageing was defined through pensions and the welfare policy. Retirement, exit from the workforce, has been used as a social as well as a financial category through which a new social space is constructed for older adults. The defining features of this space have, since the inception of the welfare state, centred on dependency as a result of physical and mental decline, plus the primacy of child care over the needs of adult groups. Adult ageing has thus been conceived as a burden on other productive, or potentially productive, parts of the population. Evidence for this view can be found in Beveridge's (1942) original document *Social Insurance and Allied Services*, on which much of the post-war consensus on health and social care was based: 'It is dangerous', he stated, 'to be in any way lavish to old age until adequate provision has been assured for all other vital needs, such as the prevention of disease and the adequate nutrition of the young' (quoted in Wilson 1991: 39).

A number of writers have shown that increased dependency, and the subsequent burdensomeness of older people on production, is by no means an inevitable consequence of ageing (Townsend 1981; Phillipson 1982; Walker 1986). In particular, Townsend (1981, 1986) has expanded on the view that dependency is socially constructed. He has proposed that this structured dependency occurs though the way that elders are systematically excluded from the working population through retirement policy, the poverty that results for the majority of the aged population, the institutionalization of a minority of older people, which then comes to stand for the majority, and restrictions that are then placed on the expected domestic and community roles made available in later life. One of the consequences of structured dependency would be that disengagement by older people from the rest of society is seen as functional, and that rather than investing in services to support an active later life, 'policies of non interference would be a greater kindness', leading to 'minimalist solutions to their problems' (Townsend 1986: 18, 19). This is despite evidence (Wilson 1991) that rather than being 'downhill all the way', as policy and provision tends to assume, the character of decline in later life is more accurately characterized as a 'terminal drop'. This means that the majority of older people are able to maintain physical and intellectual functioning right up to the final months of life.

Policy assumptions of dependency and decline are reflected in the services that have been made available to older people. Thus, Phillipson and Walker (1986: 281) note a 'Tendency to ghettoise work with the old, often placing it in the hands of the lowest paid and least trained.' Although the priorities of later life might be quite different from those of other phases of the lifecourse, these authors have observed that professionals tend to 'interpret and channel these demands (of older people) into acceptable and conventional forms' (Phillipson and Walker 1986: 282). Acceptability is age-structured, with the priorities of youth (as the dominant client group) and mid-adulthood (as the dominant worker group) characterized as central and other perspectives as marginal. Further, it is often assumed by helping professionals that, while their training has largely prepared them for work with children and young adults, it is an equally valid basis on which to make judgements about old age (Phillipson and Strang 1986). The dominant assumption that elders constitute a burden and possibly a threat to modern society is also reflected in the historical nature of interventions in the lives of older people considered to be vulnerable to abuse. Paradoxically, intervention (for example, under section 47 of the 1948 National Assistance Act) has traditionally been restricted to cases of self-neglect, whereby the conduct of older people has been judged to be a danger to the health or well-being of themselves or others.

IDENTITY AND THE EROSION OF THE WELFARE STATE

A problem with modernist policy, of both the free market and state-controlled types, is that while assumptions of dependency may be true for a minority of the most vulnerable adults, and this, in social problem terms, is a valid focus, the minority comes to stand for the dominant experience of ageing and influences future policy-making and public attitudes in an age-structured manner. This is not to say that differences fail to exist between these two forms. Phillipson and Biggs (1998) have argued that the identities and supportive lifestyles available to older people have moved from being relatively controlled and uniform towards a situation marked by increasing social diversity and a degree of social freedom. However, a negative aspect of such developments has been an erosion of the relative stability afforded by such forms of social structuration. Predictability in later life may have been exchanged for lifestyles that are increasingly insecure and uncertain.

It is suggested that in the initial transition from pre-modern to modern conditions, the widespread growth of wage labour led to youth being privileged over age. The reordering of productive relations that modernity brought with it, however, eventually created a new social space for old age in the form of pension and welfare provision. This space was, from the start, embued with ambivalence, as it represented both the success and humanity of modernity and a burden on productivity. It nevertheless constituted a fixed point around which the meaning of old age could cohere and be contested. And, insofar as persons will attempt to find social spaces that lend some form of predictability to everyday relationships, it made the groups in which an ageing identity could be adopted or resisted visible. Under postmodern conditions, however, this visibility has again come under threat, which Phillipson and Biggs associate with a move towards the consumption of identities and the adoption of market economies for health and welfare. Not only do these trends fragment the possibility of collective identity; they obscure the very age-related inequalities that the welfare state was intended to reduce. According to this perspective, midlifestylism based on the market only serves the interests of a minority of older adults: 'For the majority of older people, however, a move toward a consumer lifestyle seems only to promise further marginalisation as their engagement with society seems neither that of a producer nor of a consumer. At the same time the role of older people as "icons" of the welfare state, with an inalienable right to services, now seems under attack' (Phillipson and Biggs 1998: 8).

The argument here is not necessarily to defend the uniform and selective space that traditional welfare arrangements provided, but to point to the relative absence of a new legitimizing space for ageing itself. It is unclear where a stand can be made and what it is that acts as a spur to resistance. Estes *et al.* (1993) have described the opening up of 'no care zones' in systems of health and welfare, implying that there are some vulnerable adults who have been excluded from any form of support. Phillipson and Biggs (1998) extend this line of argument to indicate the development of 'no identity zones'. The notion of a 'no identity zone' suggests a social space in which the construction of a genuine sense of self is rendered impossible. The only spaces left available effectively deny the expression of an ageing identity, and to adopt an unacceptable identity is to render oneself invisible and unheard. It is suggested that the battleground has changed, from a place allotted to ageing which can be used as a point of reference and resistance, to one in which vulnerability must be disguised and identity subject to Machiavellian subterfuge. With the rolling back of welfare, the props to identity that in some way underwrote late-life concerns have also been significantly weakened. Accordingly, the hollowing out of the state is paralleled by a hollowing out of the ageing identity, a process which especially affects the old, the sick and those without private finance.

POSTMODERNITY AND WELFARE

Phillipson and Biggs's (1998) description of beleaguered identity and the insubstantiality of contemporary social spaces in the world of social welfare draws attention to the effects of wider social influences on identity formation. As modernist hegemonies, in the form of single defining projects around which identity takes shape, seem to melt away, it is unclear what forces will bind the individual to society.

Castoriades (1997: 85) indicates that the crisis of identity in contemporary society 'Consists in the fact that contemporary society no longer produces the types that had made it a society wanting itself . . . There cannot not be a crisis of the identification process, since there is no longer a cathected self-representation of society as the seat of meaning and of value, of a significant past and of a time to come.' Western capitalist societies, it is argued, have ceased to provide sufficiently robust links between the person and wider society, resulting in a lack of belonging which is not simply a matter of physical and geographic dislocation but extends to the forces that maintain identities intact. There is an absence of a persuasive narrative container, necessary if individuals or groups are to begin to find some coherence, some sense out of a mass of parts, episodes and experiences. The individual loses a sense of personal and societal continuity, which is reflected at a variety of social levels.

Mongardini (1992), for example, suggests that postmodern conditions have resulted in an inconsistency of the 'ego image' as a consequence of a loss of coherent social characteristics, so that it is easily absorbed into the process of continuous social change. An accompanying lack of historical consciousness is said to reduce a capacity for resistance. Such trends are apparent in the relationship between personal identifications and the connective structures, such as organizations and services, that bind citizens and society. Munro (1998) has described how contemporary managerial practices actively discourage a sense of belonging in the pursuit of continued organizational change. Agency tradition, loyalty and custom are no longer valued or needed under market conditions of plentiful and 'flexible' labour supply and globalization. The language of primary task has been used by Obholzer (1993) to chart a similar process taking place in health and social services. Here, the guiding principles for action, the inspiration of hope through the alleviation of illness and poverty, have been observed as subject to considerable strain with the growth of market and managerialist models of welfare. Priorities of economy and responsibility to funders have eroded the primacy of patient and client care, leaving the core reasoning and legitimised motivation of workers in these sectors confused. Nathan (1994) has indicated that the marketization of community care for adults has resulted in the widespread adoption of primitive psychological coping mechanisms, such as a rigid splitting of good from bad and a denial of negative outcomes. In this state of affairs, collusive alliances may become typical of some forms of adult care (Biggs 1994, 1998).

Higgs (1995) has proposed that arguing against ageism on the basis of the right of older people to full citizenship may have become outdated under contemporary conditions. A combination of social diversity, active consumerism and the encouragement to take greater personal responsibility for personal health and finance has eroded the value of universal welfare provision on which the notion of citizenship rested. Phillipson (1998) has similarly questioned the effects of contemporary social policy on citizenship in later life. However, here an erosion of the social connectedness occasioned by citizenship is seen as threatening to personal and collective identity.

Writers such as Baddeley (1995) and Bauman (1998) suggest that these new forms of indeterminacy have forced people to address the question of personal responsibility. Contrary to thinking dominant in the modern period, in its market and statist forms, Bauman (1998) suggests that responsibility to others occurs as a sense of obligation diminishes. Obligation, it is argued, relies on the strength of the other to extract it, and implies that once one's duty has been fulfilled and the contract completed, no further or wider claims can be made. Responsibility, on the other hand, is evoked by the weakness of the other, suggests an empathic recognition of the other and is, by comparison, open-ended. This view certainly reflects Finch's (1995) observations on informal care, which, despite attempts by right-wing policy-makers to enforce fixed familial obligation, is increasingly coming to reflect personal commitment and negotiated relationships. Baddeley (1995: 1073) suggests that 'At a time when neither individualism nor collectivism seem able to nurture individuality, the idea of an internal polity can enrich self awareness and strengthen a sense of agency in the world.'

In other words, where market welfare and state control have failed to create an adequate space for the expression of mature identity, a premium might be placed on an ability to internalize and reflect upon competing definitions and strategies. This analysis would suggest the evolution of a protected mental space, a sort of virtual test bed for moral action, not unlike the distinction between surface and hidden suggested by metaphors of the masque. Further, it would appear that in the absence of containers that are externally maintained, internal containing spaces might have to be created.

IMPLICATIONS: A NEW INDETERMINACY

If health and social care constitute an alternative space for ageing to that posed by the development of midlifestyles, it is clear that it is hardly more likely to contain environments in which a genuine sense of ageing identity can take shape. Each, although in characteristically different ways, restricts the aspects of personal identity that can be expressed. The likelihood of genuine identity statements occurring, in the sense of a joining of internal and external logics of ageing, seems remote. Rather, a mature identity would appear to be reflected through the distorting mirrors of excessive dependency or excessive autonomy. For many of the vulnerable old this would seem to hold the promise of being either controlled or ignored. Developments in social policy seem to indicate increased indeterminacy rather than increased security. The likelihood correspondingly increases that the containing spaces created by services will prove insufficiently robust either to form the basis of identity formation or as positions against which significant forms of resistance can take shape. A trajectory of personal and social congruence in which masquerade is minimized and genuine expression increased, requires that reflective social spaces open up in which the relationship between past, present and future can be examined and serve as a basis for agency. It is, however, unclear whether contemporary policy spaces can increase the possibilities for this form of coherence.

8

Policy spaces in health and welfare

POSSIBILITIES FOR REFLECTIVE AWARENESS

The description of social spaces contained in Chapter 7 has drawn attention to two of their qualities. First, social spaces can be seen as seemingly naturally occurring, yet socially constructed, arenas in which people can more easily perform some identities than others. Identity performance is a more or less unselfconscious activity under such conditions, and is closely related to common-sense reality as described in the work of Schutz (1962) and Berger and Luckman (1971). Identities which jar with the dominant expectations contained within any one social space would be difficult to perform in such a setting and subject to sanction. A persistent attempt to perform an identity that conflicted with the assumptions implicit in such a space could be described as an act of resistance (Foucault 1979). If no space can be found in which even resistive expression can take place, then one has entered a 'no identity zone' (Phillipson and Biggs 1998). Second, certain social spaces emerge as self-consciously reflective containers. That is to say, qualities of the containing space make it easier for people to stand back from the performance of everyday identities and make connections between them. They also invite the creation of new prefigurative spaces in which entirely different identities might take shape. An element particularly related to the emergence of mature imagination would be the likelihood of connecting here and now experience to the past and to possible futures and then working towards the self-conscious shaping of a social environment in which these relationships could be expressed.

People in this second type of space would be acting and thinking reflexively insofar as they became able to perform while taking into account the multiple social influences upon them. This could be thought of as an outer, horizontal form of awareness, as it increases understanding of contemporary social influences and possibilities. However, reflexivity lacks an inner, vertical dimension that is brought into being through a consideration of the psyche as layered and that different layers include possibly contradictory hopes and fears which influence consciousness. Awareness of this vertical layering and its effects on social behaviour is what is meant by being able to act and think reflectively.

An example of the first type of social space might be when professional workers and older adults automatically perform dependent and independent roles in conformity with unstated but commonly accepted health and welfare stereotypes. In the second type, the social environment would allow participants to understand and modify their behaviour at a number of levels, perhaps acknowledging that interaction contains elements of masquerade which might obscure more deep-seated concerns and desires, perhaps allowing participants to weave elements of their past and potential selves into a performance, perhaps confronting the networks of power that have previously fixed relationships and spaces. In each case there would be an invitation to progress beyond immediate surface elements.

Typically, social spaces emerge on a continuum between the first and second sorts, and in practical terms it is more helpful to understand the likelihood that any one space will facilitate reflexive and reflective awareness. Sometimes such spaces are 'artificially' created, as in the case of an overtly therapeutic group or a listening post, as described in Chapter 7. Sometimes a facilitative and containing space emerges alongside pre-existent material and social-psychological phenomena. Examples here might include existing institutions, organizational cultures and social policies which make it more rather than less likely that activity based on this form of understanding will occur. Spaces could be thought of as facilitative when the need for masquerade is reduced, and a merging of inner and outer logics informs personal agency. Primacy is assumed for an inner logic, which is nevertheless in tune with, or tuned into, external and intersubjective realities. The apprehension of social realities is thus rendered reflectively real. A social space is therefore a social and psychological reality which may or may not correspond with a particular physical environment. It is held in place by a number of factors, including the interests of powerful stakeholders, policies and regulations, political and professional ideologies. It contributes to the likelihood of a certain masquerade being performed and the possibility that deeper layers of psychological meaning can be expressed. Spaces that emerge in the field of social policy are particularly important to the mature imagination because they have come to define, in the popular mind, the shape and circumference of ageing.

POLICY AND SOCIAL SPACE

In questions of health and welfare a factor of defining importance for the shape and possibilities inherent in a social space is the environment created by social policy. Each of the three movements in Western social policy since the Second World War can be seen as an invitation to think differently about freedom of expression, and thus the ways in which people must perform to benefit. There follows a potted history of state, market and the 'new' social democratic welfarism, which highlights some of these key factors.

Under the classic welfare state (Lowe 1994) which formed the basis for post-war welfare consensus on health and social care, participation was by mandate, and freedom and security were increased through the removal of debilitating barriers to self-improvement. Thus, it was assumed that if Beveridge's (1942) five giants of want, ignorance, squalor, disease and idleness could be slain, or at least diminished in size, equality of opportunity would be increased. This model relied on state intervention legitimized by the popular vote, plus the inclusion of considerable deference to expert opinion. State intervention increased uniform support, but fuelled a myth of an emerging dependency culture (Dean and Taylor-Gooby 1992) which eventually became its undoing. Removal of barriers to self-development was perceived to increase the adoption of a dependent performance on the part of some of those who used its services.

Market models have promised participation through the hidden hand of accumulated choices. These are seen to be made by individual consumers and the injection of competitive and managerial values into services (Le Grand and Bartlett 1993). Self-expression comes to be dominated, under such an approach, by a relative ability to pick and choose provision on the basis of the best available information. The legitimacy of different participants in health and social care is conceived in terms of purchasing power, efficient provision and consumer desire, plus the elimination of vested interests. This market vision also requires that a rigid distinction be made between the public sphere of the market and private and collective loyalties. This is deemed necessary to ensure unbiased competition (Bauman 1995), but also gives rise to coercive approaches to caring obligations. These forces eventually fragment welfare environments and result in increased uncertainty and an unravelling of established relations, resulting in unsustainable levels of social exclusion.

Social democratic conceptions of health and social care have valued participative decision-taking by stakeholders (Blair 1996). Stakeholders are seen to include a large number of groups and interests who will affect or be affected by emergent social policy, and spreads consultation on it beyond immediate users, providers and purchasers, to include specific pressure and interest groups and less specifically defined social and geographic communities. A key motivation behind social policy of this type is to decrease social exclusion (Jordan 1996) so as to re-establish a commonly held social project with which all members of society can identify (MacPherson 1997). Social inclusion is seen to depend upon citizens accepting certain responsibilities as well as rights, and in this respect draws heavily on ideas of communitarianism (Etzioni 1997). Valid performances tend to depend on an ability or willingness to take part in various mechanisms for partnership, introducing concerns about the degree to which potential participants have the capacity to be included.

Under each of these movements in social policy, the space available for legitimate social performance has changed shape, and invites different possibilities for mature identity. They also configure the value of health and welfare services in different ways and raise diverse questions about the explanatory value of primary task.

CHALLENGES TO PRIMARY TASK

The concept of primary task, which is heavily reliant upon the notion of a single and determining goal for social activity in organizations, is challenged by each of the policy spaces outlined above. It is perhaps best suited to a unitary model, as exemplified by statist intervention in health and welfare. A single core policy, while always something of a fiction, is most easily identified under conditions where provision is uniform and universal. It is easier to articulate a formal 'work task' against which alternative conceptions of function and activity can be judged. The implications of such shaping can be felt throughout a social system as provision takes on the standard and 'total' character exemplified by Goffman's (1961) study of asylums and Townsend's (1963) work on the institutionalization of older people. Mechanisms, both formal and informal, arise to maintain behavioural conformity and categorize dissent as deviation. Difficulty is experienced in acknowledging the legitimacy of claims to difference along, among others, lines of ethnicity (Patel 1990), gender (Bernard and Meade 1993) and disability (Morris 1991). Here, the primary task model can be used to understand distinctions between what a system has been set up to do, and the uses and contested spaces that emerge as it develops. The point is less that weaknesses of an account based on primary task lie in the privileging of one definition of activity over another (although it tends to do this as well), than that it assumes an underlying state of stability within the whole system. It is possible to talk in terms of primary task because it can be assumed that the task is relatively fixed. It can thus act as a stable point of reference in relation to which people can take a stand of agreement or resistance. If, however, the system is itself in a state of flux, notions of primary task tend to break down.

Challenges to the primacy of one guiding task exist in both the market and social democratic models of health and welfare policy. Market conceptions of welfare have been part of a wider attempt to engineer a shift in social behaviour away from organized collectivism, and it might be argued collective altruism, towards a system driven by competition and individualism. They also place economic priorities of efficiency and accountability to funders over professional ethics and notions of care for its own sake (Caputo 1988). If welfare is seen, for example, as creating dependency and a drain on the national economy, a core goal of policy becomes the reduction of these costs, which have then to become part and parcel of each interaction between professional helpers and people who require services. One of the issues in this area is whether it is possible to graft principles and solutions essentially generated for other social priorities on to welfare systems, without raising a series of new problems. Here, the imposition of market economic solutions to problems that consist largely of human distress and vulnerability leads to conflicting notions of primary task. On the one hand the task would be to alleviate need and on the other to reduce costs to other parts of society, thus reducing the services available for the first task. So incompatible work priorities come to inhabit the same policy space. The problem in terms of primary task is that the ideology in question is intended to achieve quite different results from those suggested by the original institutional task, and a struggle for dominance results.

The social-democratic emphasis on stakeholding also destabilizes the notion of a single primary task. Here, multiple and competing definitions and priorities need to be taken explicitly into account within the policy arena. Thus it is difficult to arrive at one morally ascendant definition of task. There are, of course, contradictions and tensions within the social-democratic project, in that the antidote to social exclusion is seen in finding a task that can, in its ideal form, include all interests. Pragmatically, however, the process of achieving a maximum number of adherents requires attention to the negotiated and contingent qualities of decision-making. The notion of primacy has therefore to change from an explicit and single work task to a higher-level objective of creating a space within which negotiated solutions can be found. In other words, it has moved from an explicit policy concern with content to one that attempts to create and sustain the conditions under which participation can take place. The move towards recognizing a multiplicity of agendas, and the idea that policy might best be conceived as a force that facilitates process rather than content, challenges the notion of primacy.

Lawrence's (1977) attempt to configure multiple primary tasks does not help here: first, because he mostly describes misunderstandings or accommodations to a task which is ill-defined; and second, because to suggest multiple primary tasks contradicts the essence of primacy itself. Semantically speaking, there can either be a primary task which dominates or multiple tasks, but not both.

This debate on primacy versus multiplicity highlights the family resemblances between changes in policy and the proposition that we are

living in postmodern times. This is particularly the case when professional and service user identities are discussed. Both market and social-
democratic approaches to welfare reflect trends that have previously been
identified with a move from conditions of modernity to postmodernity,
and it is to that debate that we now return.

IDENTITIES, PARTNERSHIP AND POSTMODERNITY

That adult service systems exist under conditions of continued flux and
uncertainty has been noted on both sides of the Atlantic (Estes *et al.*,
1993; Howe 1994; Leonard 1997). A discussion of policy as shaping social
space highlights the point that change is not simply structural in its
effects, but also influences how identities are managed between service
users and helping professionals and between different professional groups.
Debates on user participation and interprofessionalism are two areas in
which traditional positions have become contested and the opportunities
for new relationships are most apparent. In this context identity becomes
an important crossroads between the experience of self, day-to-day communication and expectations arising from social policy. In this sense, the
study of identities that different professions, players, stakeholders and
interests adopt serves as a bridge to understanding the relationship
between the personal and broader social and political forces. The permeability of these identities – in other words, how far the barriers between
various groups can be reduced – and whether this is perceived as desirable would influence how participants behave towards each other and
their responsiveness to policy change.

Partnership, in both its interprofessional and participative aspects,
presents a considerable challenge to the performance of adult identity
under conditions of modernity. Modernity refers, in this context, to a
society in which boundaries are relatively impermeable and identities
are more or less fixed, as are expectations on the conduct of relationships
between groups and individuals. There can be little doubt that much of
the traditional identity of professional groupings rests on what can now
be identified as 'modern' foundations. Medicine and nursing, for example,
have drawn heavily on technical/scientific knowledge to justify their
expert status, while social work has been closely identified with notions
of universality and equity. Both health and welfare professions have been
seen as part and parcel of a great movement for progress characteristic of
much of the twentieth century. Under modern conditions, professional
boundaries and a clear distinction between helper and helped would be
key to keeping service systems stable and predictable.

Postmodernity leads to a questioning of these foundations by point-
ing to the arbitrariness of professional divisions, the unforeseen risks

associated with scientific progress and the possibility of choosing identities that may not be governed by ascribed roles and hierarchies. It marks a shift towards a much more fluid state of affairs, in which certain identities might be chosen in order to enter particular relationships with others, but then discarded as other situations and opportunities become available. Similarly, boundaries between groups become more permeable, allowing greater awareness of interconnectedness and movement between institutional systems (a greater awareness, for example, that chief executives can also be patients and that service users with disabilities have active lives and identities independent of medical conditions).

This postmodern perspective suggests that identity is no longer a stable phenomenon and that the hierarchies that aim to fix relationships, such as that between 'senior' professions and professions related to them, and that between those who control the allocation of services and those who need and receive them, are breaking down. Many of the trends associated with health and welfare reform would resonate with this analysis, at least at the level of policy on the relationship between professions. Developments such as the blurring of distinctions between medicine and advanced nursing practice and the movement of staff from a variety of professional backgrounds into management positions could be interpreted as evidence of postmodern change. Indeed, increased emphasis given to monitoring and coordination, multiprofessionalism and user participation would also suggest new spaces in which users and professionals work together, created by the breakdown of established boundaries. In other words, contemporary service trends are prefigurative in that they make some relationships more likely to emerge than others. Under postmodern conditions, one would expect positions to become flexible and interchangeable. The identities of people who make up the system would change, chameleon-like, depending on the situation in which they found themselves. Service users become persons in need in one context, experts in the consumption of services in another and decision-makers in yet another. Professional workers similarly become specialists, advocates, purchasers, providers and consumers of services depending on their circumstances.

UTOPIAN POSSIBILITIES

Crook *et al.* (1992) have outlined a process characteristic of moves from modernity and into postmodernity, which immediately suggests parallels with trends towards interprofessionalism and user participation. They indicate that organizational and professional cultures and identities mutate from a situation of differentiation through hyperdifferentiation and towards dedifferentiation. Differentiation refers to a separating out of particular groups. These might include the professions of medicine, nursing, psychology, social work and so on. Differentiation also describes a clearer distinction, emergent between professionals and users. Differentiation allows the development of particular groupings of expertise and closer communication within groups with the same specialist knowledge. Professional identities come to be based on the increasing specification of identifiably distinct and differentiated patient or client groups. However, as these processes gather pace, distinctions become hyperdifferentiated. Specialisms become so marked and so circumscribed that it is difficult, even for members of the same professional group, to communicate meaningfully. A consequence of this hyperdifferentiated specialization is that it is as easy to communicate with someone in a completely different field, or in markedly different circumstances, as it is to restrict communication to an exclusively intraprofessional discourse. Communication then becomes 'dedifferentiated'. This would mean that professionals begin to share ideas across 'modern' professional boundaries, and it becomes easier for users and workers to share in decision-making.

This process of diversification and recombination would suggest new opportunities for users and professionals to work together in the space created by the breakdown of old divisions, an increased permeability of boundaries and openness to alternative perspectives. Moves towards user participation and interprofessionalism might both reflect and contribute to this momentum, away from old certainties and towards a situation that is more ambiguous and in many cases more ambivalent as well. User participation suggests an increasing permeability for boundaries between professionals and non-professionals, while interprofessionalism presents a similar challenge to distinctions within the professional arena.

Interprofessionalism and participation

A striking feature of research on interprofessionalism and participation is that it is fragmentary and small in scale. Beckingham (1997), in her review of US and Canadian literature, has called this the 'Here's what we do at our university or in this service setting' approach to collaboration. Unsurprisingly, perhaps, this coexists with an absence, relative to other fields of applied research, of conceptual models and theoretical frameworks. The frameworks that are being used fall into two categories. First, there are approaches arising directly from a particular position in the service system. These would include an 'empowerment' perspective, as promoted by users themselves (Croft and Beresford 1992; Morris 1992; Town et al. 1997) and their allies (Ward and Mullander 1991; Stevens 1993), which generally describes barriers to active participation. By contrast, writers from a broadly 'managerialist' perspective (Øvretveit 1993; Nocon 1994; Mitchell and Coats 1997) have focused on how service systems work and can be developed. A second group of approaches has arisen from particular theoretical positions. Most notable here are workers using a psychodynamic framework (Woodhouse and Pengelly 1991; Stokes 1994), a systems approach (Rawson 1994) and a functionalist approach (Øvretveit *et al.* 1997), although in this last example the model is often assumed rather than explicit.

There appears, however, to be relatively little dialogue across these positional and theoretical boundaries, nor between different positions and interests. Biggs (1993b: 153) has, for example, noted in a review of partnership issues that: 'Whilst there are debates on both interprofessional collaboration and user participation, there is almost no literature on the relationship between the two.' The reader is left with an impression that writers in this field exist on the boundaries of a number of intersecting interests. Practitioners write up their collaborative projects. Activists set out their stalls. Theorists periodically turn their attention to its continuing development. As a whole, the discussion of interprofessionalism and user voice reproduces characteristics of its field of study insofar as it is partial and frequently consists of atomized instances and explanations. In this context, Katz (1996) has noted that while gerontology has from its inception involved a variety of disciplines, it consists of groups that live side-by-side rather than in meaningful dialogue. There is very little genuine sharing of perspectives or attempt at merger. Partnership is, in this sense, everyone's relative but no one's child.

Despite these discontinuities in the literature, it is possible to draw out key areas of agreement. To begin with, both participation and interdisciplinarity are viewed as positive developments that in some way improve service delivery. Second, a paradigm shift towards shared definitions of service situations is required if positive change is to take place. Third, effective partnership requires a negotiated balance between the special contributions of each partner. Finally, identification with an overarching goal that is greater than any individual contribution acts to bind participants together. However, it is unclear how far these common factors may simply mark out the value judgements of the field itself. They often have the feel of being reactions to problems of coordination that are tacit, rather than explicitly drawn.

A focus on older people as specified partners in interprofessional care is limited. Much of the literature takes a generic position towards user groups, to which can be added significant contributions from the fields of mental health and disability. Work that refers specifically to older people includes: Biggs (1993b), who used examples from primary and community care services for older people and their carers; Sparkes's (1994) study of professional attitudes towards older people within an interprofessional context; Evers *et al.*'s (1994) review of interprofessional work with old and disabled people; Myers and MacDonald's (1996) description of social worker evaluations of user involvement, which draws on work with older people; Beckingham's (1997) paper on interdisciplinary health care teamwork in the care of the elderly; and Camara's (1997) description of interdisciplinary elderly care in Brazil. Common themes include: the older person (in this case, as a nominated user or as an informal carer) as expert in the consumption of care, its coordination and quality; the tendency for attitudes to older people and their needs to be influenced by professional background and forms of organization; and the tendency for gerontology to be naturally interdisciplinary by virtue of the complexity and multi-faceted experience of health and ageing.

Beckingham (1997: 19) observes that interdisciplinary collaboration is often interpreted 'to mean that boundaries of disciplines will become increasingly blurred and members will exchange roles and responsibilities according to the needs of the situation.' Certainly, literature on participation seems to assume the adoption of multiple roles and identities, such that users may become recipients of care at one moment, co-workers the next and quality assessors in yet another. Such observations are tempered by Rawson (1994), who considers that the establishment of internal markets in health care has made professions increasingly rivalrous and prone to defensiveness. Rather than blurring boundaries, the extra stress associated with competition makes professionals retreat to more rigid identities. The complexity of participative and interprofessional frameworks may be owing in part to policy trends which are apparently pulling in different directions (Biggs 1997a, b). First, unifying tendencies towards general management and quality control tend to merge operational identities. Second, diversifying tendencies towards user participation and the appreciation of individual need tend to foster a fragmentation of pre-existing systems. If identities are to respond flexibly to these new conditions, participants might need to experience autonomy within a containing and supportive structure, which would have a strong performative element (Latimer 1997). This structure would be able to sustain a crucial balance between the blurring of roles and the recognition of specialist expertise. Trends towards the establishment of multiple identities help to keep such systems afloat in that, identity wise, participants can keep their options open. Similarly, a migration to the boundaries of systems and a concentration on boundary management protects identity through distance. Examples of boundary management include inspection and quality control as well as interprofessional collaboration. In each case the focus of activity has moved away from what is going on within any one context, and towards negotiations across or between contexts and sectors.

Expert consumption and para-professionalism

Where partnership has led to a blurring of traditional role relationships, it may also lead to the opening up of new spaces in which to exercise the mature imagination. Key to understanding this possibility is the degree to which, during the performance of identity in these spaces, expression is promoted or hidden.

One notion that repeatedly arises in this literature is that of the adult service user as expert in some way. Thus, Evers *et al.* (1994) have proposed that older people and their carers are expert in a variety of ways: on themselves, on their requirements and in negotiating the vagaries of service provision. Recognition of users as expert consumers (Biggs 1993b) would provide an active legitimizing role which might form the basis of a more equal communication with professionals. Rawson (1994) similarly identifies the 'client as an active partner' in some aspects of the inter-professional process. This, he says, is most apparent as 'articulation work', whereby the efforts of team members must be given a coherent form, rather than becoming a collection of unrelated inputs. The user or carer becomes the one person who maintains a sense of continuity, experiences the gaps and thus holds valuable information on the quality of service.

It has been argued by Miles (1994) that while progress has been slow, new arrangements for community care have opened an opportunity for participation in decision-making that had not previously been available. The development of 'elderly forums' and formal mechanisms for support and consultation has provided a space within which being someone who uses services carries a positive and active connotation. Miles has been active in facilitating the position of carers of older people as advisors in the reorganization of service systems across existing service boundaries. Similar work in psychiatric settings (Steinberg 1992) indicates that inter-professional working may be especially fertile ground for the involvement of users as properly informed participants. This, he suggests, is due to the need for a style in which professionals learn to help to manage aspects of each other's work without taking it over.

The quest for expert partnership has extended to residential settings. Means and Smith (1994) have noted that while market models of care have tended to emphasize empowerment through the right of 'exit', they have also led to a growth in regulation and quality control in which people can directly participate. For example, van Geen (1997) reports on a 'measure and discuss' method which promotes empowerment though the regular use of focus groups. Here an external body collaborates with residents in presenting their analysis of care quality and in monitoring improvements. Opportunities for using older people as 'lay inspectors' or 'undercover grannies', in other words as consultants to registration and inspection teams, have recently been revived by Boateng (1997).

This focus on expertness has been closely related to the view that the users of services can take on some of the skills used by trained workers. They can, in other words, become para-professionals. Thus, Bond (1992) has argued that one of the consequences of the introduction of care management and coordination roles has been a growing respect of carers as the working partners of professional helpers. Twigg and Aitkin (1993) also identified co-working as one of four forms of carer–professional relationship, which may now be privileged by policy trends. Para-professionalism refers to co-opting the carer into a similar role to the professional worker in some areas, and includes the transfer of skills and specific training being developed for the carer. It is contended that this would enhance and legitimize carer status and might eventually lead to a situation described by Øvretveit (1997) as 'co-servicing'. However, such trends have also been greeted with caution. Biggs (1993a) has argued that alliances based on tasks shared between care managers and informal carers can lead to collusion that can exclude the person being cared for. In addition, it may become increasingly difficult for the co-opted person to express his or her separate needs and identity. Forbes and Sashidharan (1997) point out that while the inclusion of users in the organization and delivery of services has been welcomed by planners, academics and practitioners, it brings the danger that users will be incorporated into existing systems and lose their ability to challenge them.

If, as has been suggested above, trends towards interprofessionalism and participation have contributed to the opening up of new spaces in which to perform welfare identities, partners as expert and as para-professional would appear to be strong candidates. They tie in well both with the market ideology of autonomy and choice and with the 'new' social democratic demand for stakeholding and negotiation through participation. However, both also rely on the user of services becoming ever closer, in terms of identity, to those who work in a particular service. Expertness ensures a place at a table that pre-exists, and has a shape that has already been agreed. One performs as an expert among all the other experts. While it allows the possibility of reflexive engagement with service processes, this should not be mistaken for the expression of a reflective engagement with deeper psychological processes. How far one is able to be oneself in partnership, rather than simply servicing the agendas of others, is rarely explicitly addressed. Similarly, para-professionalization says little about the inner logic of the adult psyche. Instead, it ensures conformity to a different intersubjective world, that of professionality. In both cases the invitation, extended under the banner of partnership, is to become 'one of us', to enter the space of professional concerns. It is certainly an active role, but, as we have seen, activity is not necessary the ally of critical reflective space.

The utopian scenarios sketched out in these spaces exhibit a tendency to assume that participants are well, solvent and articulate. The consumer of health and welfare has thus to masquerade as simultaneously independent and autonomous as well as in distress. By the drawing of users into human service systems, it is argued, they can achieve a recognition and status that would not otherwise be available to them. However, this process would also tend to disguise imbalances in power between parties in its attempt to define a common project in which all stakeholders can be usefully employed. What is unclear is where the existential concerns of age might fit in such a scenario, if it is based upon improving services in their existing forms. If there are no substantive means of addressing hidden or vertical levels of meaning, then partnership simply approximates a wider, rather than deeper, exercise in quality control. It is also unclear how people whose conditions inhibit participation find a place within this scheme of things. The question of where to locate people whose circumstances, conduct or desires may not fit into this utopian space is discussed below.

DYSTOPIAN POSSIBILITIES

The view described above is at once familiar and puzzlingly awry as a description of contemporary health and welfare. If this is a utopian vision of the postmodern welfare state, there are also discordant and distinctly dystopian possibilities lurking beneath its celebration of surface relationships. Problems arise as a result of what initially appear to be the 'free floating' identities that postmodern thinkers have suggested, but on closer inspection exist in a closely circumscribed social space. A central feature of the response to fragmentation and changeability, that it is no longer certain where boundaries should be drawn and how stable and reliable those boundaries are, is to attempt a premature closure and again to fix identity and make it predictable. Under such conditions, felt uncertainty would affect both professional and user positions, provoking a defensive retrenchment and the erection of rigid boundaries. Using the example of social work, Howe (1994: 513) describes this growing uncertainty in the following way: 'A child of modernity, social work now finds itself in a postmodern world, uncertain whether or not there are any deep and unwavering principles which define the essence of its character and hold it together as a coherent enterprise.' Further, the nature of citizenship, a concept closely linked to that of participation and to hearing the user's voice, has also been subjected to a destabilizing attack. Citizenship 'has moved from being an embodiment of universal social rights to a much more narrow conception . . . This shift is in part the product of changes in social structure which have led individuals to stress their difference from one another rather than their (common) identity' (Higgs 1995: 536).

So what is happening to those boundaries that describe legitimacy? While there is movement towards fluidity, is there not also a sequestration of experience that Giddens (1991) has warned us about, and that in

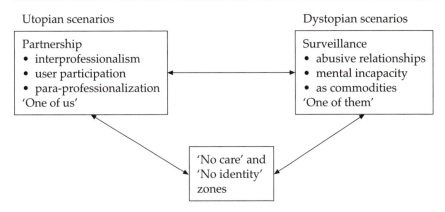

Figure 8.1 Contemporary policy spaces.

psychodynamic terms would be thought of as a splitting off of incompatible conflicts of identity? (Nathan 1994) Two developments in contemporary social policy give some indication of the dystopian spaces that are taking shape around those who will not or cannot become active participants in partnership. First, there has been a growing concern with adults as the subjects of abuse and an accompanying preoccupation with surveillance. The growth of concern about adult protection in the USA (Baumhover and Beall 1996) and the UK and Australasia (Kingston and Penhale 1995) marks an interesting case study in the development of new social spaces in which overt and tacit agendas can be identified. Second, there has been a perceived need to define the conditions under which users fail in their mental capacity. In other words, a debate has emerged over how to legitimize absence from other legitimizing spaces.

THE OBJECTS OF SURVEILLANCE

One consequence of the 'hollowing out' of the state (Rhodes 1995) that accompanied marketization has been the distancing of workers and service users from each other. This includes a migration away from contact with the complex and emotionally disturbing material associated with direct care and towards the regulation of spaces in which informal or privatized care takes place. A number of concrete policy initiatives can, in retrospect, be seen as contributing to a change of practice in this direction. These include the inspection of services delivered outwith the state (Brammer 1994), the development of community supervision (Atkinson 1996) and an increased interest in adult abuse and protection (Biggs *et al.* 1995). Each of these developments has decreased the role of direct care and increased the role of some form of monitoring conduct. In other words, as part of the dystopian underbelly of contemporary welfare, the new space emerging for non-participative adults is as the objects of surveillance.

This space is Foucauldian in character, such that coercive mechanisms permeate social systems beyond actual, physical, institutions. Techniques of control, it appears, are being 'broken down into flexible methods of control, which may be transferred and adapted . . . [as] centres of observation disseminated throughout society' (Foucault 1977: 211–12).

Followers of Foucault, such as Porter (1997), have linked surveillance to the promotion of holistic care. Holism is part and parcel of increased surveillance into the minutiae of daily life. It is argued that, on the one hand, practitioners are encouraged to see users as rounded individuals, while, on the other, holism brings increasingly more of an individual's behaviour and personality under professional control. Brammer and Biggs (1998) have argued that a similar process of ever broader and more inclusive definitions of abusive behaviour serves a similar function in the case of elder protection. In Foucault's work, a process is described whereby conventional values are in flux, and professional discourses emerge to interpenetrate the evolution of new commonsensual understandings of normality. As a newly defined social problem takes shape, disciplines emerge and 'swarm' around it, making sense of it and defining its parameters (Foucault 1977). Further, Foucault (1979: 86) indicated that 'power is tolerable only on condition that it mask a substantial part of itself. Its success is proportional to its ability to hide its own mechanisms.' Observations such as these have provoked Penna and O'Brien (1996) to note that modern health and welfare institutions often operate according to logics that are at extreme variance from their normative humanitarian concerns.

It emerges, from this analysis, that the creation of a new social space is very much a dynamic process which coheres over time and at some point comes together. Elements that had previously developed independently might begin to 'make sense' in new ways as spaces becomes established. However, the underlying processes of control that lend shape to any one space may not be the same as its products, nor an overt rationale that would usually be employed to justify it. The processes and effects of such systems may be hidden from both those who operate within them and those upon whom they are employed.

Elder abuse had been identified as a social problem in both the USA (O'Malley *et al.* 1979) and the UK (Eastman 1984), but until the 1990s had only provoked a policy and practice response only in the USA (Pillemer and Wolf 1986). This suggests that the 'discovery' of abuse may be the product of particular social and historical conditions. These conditions would lend a coherence and meaning to abuse that would not otherwise be available to it. Such coherence goes beyond the commendable humanitarian reasoning that demands that adults be able to live their lives free from intimidation and exploitation. It indicates that an understanding of abuse has been shaped by particular political, professional and policy concerns. In the UK, formal recognition of this 'new' social problem occurred contemporaneously with a policy initiative, the implementation of the 1990 NHS and Community Care Act, which included moves, through the adoption of care management, to engineer a privatized welfare economy with an emphasis on obligatory care by relatives. Care management was introduced as a specialist method of coordinating privatized support to an informal carer at minimum cost. A common aim of such policies in English-speaking countries has been to transfer financial and caring responsibility for dependent adults away from the collective and on to individual families. While USA literature available at the time of adoption in the UK and Australia had identified a variety of case management models (see Kanter 1988; Austin and O'Connor 1989; Moxley 1989), it is equally clear that policy-makers identified a version of case management which emphasized its role in facilitating the development of a welfare market, rather than direct intervention.

This model, in terms of rationale and orientation, did not fit well with other trends in welfare practice. In other words, while this technology solved a policy problem of how to engineer a privatized welfare economy, it made little sense for front-line workers, until that time engaged in direct service provision. Further, its signature was one of indirectness, assessment and monitoring. It existed as a solution at the fiscal level which required a problem at the level of face-work to lend it coherence.

The problem of adult abuse had reached professional salience at a time when the relationship between formal and informal care was being restructured. The role of professional workers and the nature of informal care were both contested and in a state of considerable flux. The absence of a formal mechanism for enforcing informal care-giving, which is at root a voluntary activity, was problematic for such a policy and has arguably found resolution through an emphasis on forms of abuse perpetrated by carers on service users (Biggs 1996). Further, the changes provoked a crisis of primary task, noted earlier, for professional carers, who found their direct care roles being replaced by the assessment and monitoring entailed by care management. This sudden concern for the safety and financial security of vulnerable adults legitimized a powerful role for welfare professionals within the otherwise bleak landscape created by community care policy.

It is not, then, that community care has made us more aware of forms of adult abuse, but that abuse gives meaning to care in the community, which had lost its primary task. Before the 'discovery' of abuse, technologies such as case management were, at least at the level of practice, the welfare equivalent of a solution looking for a problem. Case management had been introduced to reduce welfare expenditure and was out of sympathy with the existing task of direct care. Monitoring for adult abuse filled a vacuum at the heart of community care policy, giving it a coherence it previously lacked. Abuse provides the excuse for this invasion of the private sphere, a shift from consent to coercion and from support to surveillance. Contemporary awareness of adult abuse may radically change the space in which adult services exist, and combines with agreement in the UK (Decalmer and Glendenning 1993) and the USA (Baumhover and Beall 1996) that interprofessionality will become increasingly important as services respond to abuse. In this, adult protective services can be expected to follow trends in child protection towards interprofessional collaboration and investigatory technique (Hallett and Birchall 1992). The persuasiveness of the 'abuse' phenomenon lies in its ability to tap into a number of discourses in the care of older people, combining reference to longstanding critiques of institutional care, ageism and a search for higher-status professional identities and collaborations.

There is another snake in the postmodern utopia, and it concerns the question of what to do with people who cannot or will not participate. This trend is reflected in activities of the UK Law Commission and in the Lord Chancellor's (1997) consultation paper on mental incapacity entitled *Who Decides?* The initiative constitutes an attempt to achieve a legally binding test of capacity, when it would be in the best interests of the individual adult in receipt of care to have decisions taken for him or her and the conditions and qualities of persons given the general authority to act reasonably under such circumstances. The debate has expanded to include the public law protection of people at risk, which includes the awarding of powers to professionals to investigate suspected cases of abuse. These developments therefore consider when an adult can be judged unable to make his or her own decisions, a consideration which has been linked to the granting of adult protective powers.

Viewed in the light of policy movement in the direction of partnership, the debate on mental capacity can be seen as a search for a place for non-participants. It solves the problem of how to locate people who have become the shadow side of the great stakeholding project, and objectifies the conditions under which adults can legitimately be excused from entering that space. A problem here lies in the possibility that being mentally incapacitated is not the only criterion for social inclusion, exclusion or exploitation. First, Podnieks (1992), for example, has argued that abused older people are in fact tough, stoical survivors, while other writers (in Biggs *et al.* 1995) have drawn attention to the myth, commonly held among caring professionals, that abused adults are dependent on their abusers, whereas evidence points to the abuser often being dependent, emotionally or materially, on the victim. Second, Davis (1996) has pointed out that empowerment philosophy, which would include moves towards partnership, is more a system of values than a model of mental health and illness, and cannot in itself act as a framework for understanding and working with disturbed people. An exclusive positioning of relationships in terms of partnership might thereby eclipse the space set aside for less tractable problems, such as illness, poverty and mental disability. These observations are reminiscent of Miller and Gwynne's (1972) finding that professionals might set unrealistic goals for people who are in reality vulnerable and frail, and Gubrium and Wallace's (1990) parody of the uncritical application of activity theory regardless of the health status of older residents.

There is a danger, in other words, that new spaces have been created on the assumption that there is actually very little wrong with people in receipt of care and that they can therefore be treated 'like anyone else'. If the climate of care fosters such expectations, which would tend to ignore real disabilities, users are being set up to fail, for rather than only the disability being seen, as had occurred under modernist welfare (Oliver 1990), the disability has now been occluded and is hardly seen at all. Just as a postmodern reliance on consumer identity has been used to eclipse the limits set by an ageing body and finitude, the partnership space for welfare tends to disguise the perception of core needs. This line of argument suggests that such aspects of identity would, therefore, be avoided or denied within the legitimizing spaces that are themselves emerging in reaction to the passive/illness/disengagement roles traditionally attributed to older people. The debate on incapacity would seem to give some validation to Phillipson and Biggs's (1998) 'no identity' hypothesis. With the rolling back of welfare, the props to identity that in some way underwrote late-life concerns, have also been significantly weakened. The 'new' identities on offer, of midlifestylism and partnership, either fail to address or are based on a denial of actual dependence, and leave little space in which these needs can be voiced. Policy on abuse, increasingly associated with incapacity, defines a space where victims can be legitimately observed if they cannot find a place as active and participating. According to this view, the hollowing out of the state is paralleled by a hollowing out of the ageing identity.

IMPLICATIONS: SPACES IN WHICH TO GROW OLD?

It would seem from the above that health and welfare services, a traditional point of reference for the later stages of an ageing identity, have been subject to periods of considerable flux, and that these processes are throwing up new spaces in which identities can be performed. It is argued that ageing has been split into two separate spaces, one concerning partnership and another concerning vulnerability. Both spaces exhibit considerable ambivalence as to the likelihood that genuine self-expression could be sustained within them. Participation suggests the beginnings of negotiation around shared definitions of caring space, but a wish for uniformity in social inclusion might disguise real differences in power to determine the shape of such spaces. The doppelganger of partnership, as expressed in the debate over capacity and surveillance, on the one hand begins to define a space that allows legitimate exclusion and on the other reverts to a very modern notion of the removal of constraints (the abuse by others) to increase personal freedom. It appears, however, that as part and parcel of this latter development, ageing has become the subject of intensified monitoring and control.

This is not to say that markers for self-expressive social spaces are failing to emerge, although they are often in vague and prefigurative forms. Leonard (1997) has pointed out that contemporary health and social care is both emancipatory and a means of social regulation. It 'objectifies and controls while *at the same time* it represents a commitment to human caring' (Leonard 1997: 94, italics in original). Thus, a seat at the table of partnership includes the possibility of a say in the process of change, and freedom from abuse is a fundamental starting block from which to engage in personal and social agency as well as the negative implications noted in the previous section.

Perhaps, in the light of this contradictory nature, it is necessary to revisit the debate on midlifestyle and the creation of age-specific communities. The core problem with midlifestylism as a means to achieving a meaningful mature identity is that it is based as much on denial as it is on the recognition of the priorities of later life itself. It has picked up the message that successful ageing depends on maintenance, while ignoring the changed priorities that also emerge. It has embraced a horizontal multiplicity of surface identities without embracing deeper layers of self-expression. Thus, retirement communities, as material manifestations of extended midlife, have tended to exhibit difficulty in dealing with the increasing frailty that comes with advancing age, resulting in an ejection of members who fail to maintain strict criteria for physical and mental capacity (Latimer 1998). Researchers have noted a tendency to pervert the protective space that such communities provide by denigrating other, largely inner-city, communities, which Kastenbaum (1993) has associated with a tacit racism, and Laws (1995) with a sanctioning of similar attitudes to younger generations and elders who wish to associate with them.

This should not, however, eclipse the possibilities for personal renewal held within other ways of using living space as props to development of a mature identity. Peace *et al.* (1997), for example, note three interrelated shifts in such provision which have opened it up as an intergenerational space, while increasing the power to grow old with autonomy and security. They include within this list a move towards the explicit recognition that there are multiple stakeholders, that dependency is socially constructed and that institutional climate can play a significant role in both increasing or reducing it, and recognition of the positive value of shared decision-taking at a local level between workers and residents. Typical of such developments would be Extra Care's experiments with age-based communities in the UK's West Midlands (Biggs *et al.* 1998). Here members have often lived in the surrounding working-class area for much of their lives, and see movement into the retirement community as a new tenancy rather than primarily a move into supportive care. In the Netherlands, Baars and Thomese (1994) have noted the rapid growth of communes as positive alternatives to traditional ideas on ageing. The authors report that 'Communes provide for members an opportunity to share and give meaning to a phase of life that presently offers many unexplored possibilities' (Baars and Thomese 1994: 348). These communes are small in scale, consisting on average of between 10 and 20 members, while the age of the membership varies between 50 and 85 years old. Unlike retirement communities, these spaces often include people from different socio-economic groups. Peeters and Woldringh (1988) have suggested that communes occupy a position midway between functional networks, such as occur in clubs and institutions, and informal relationships, such as exist in friendships and families. Considerable time appears to be spent in a continued negotiation of intimacy, involvement with the collective and boundaries with surrounding communities.

These new developments seem to offer a compromise between 'ageing in place' as described by Callahan and Lansbery (1997) and Minkler (1996) and closed, age-homogeneous environments. Ageing in place refers to areas or local communities with a naturally occurring ageing membership, such as a particular district or housing complex, an advantage of which is that residents remain connected to wider social interaction. A recent research interest in the value of friendship (Phillipson 1997; Pahl and Spencer 1998) rather than locality as a basis for community life would support the value of communal 'communities of interest' as a basis for late-life development. These associations, like the activities of the communards described above, would seem to promise the possibility of both social connection and a space for reflective ageing. At best these developments are being shaped by older adults themselves and constitute an attempt to tolerate the ambiguity between the mature imagination and newly emerging social spaces. They are perhaps prefigurative of environments that do not lose themselves in the closed logic of midlifestylism and form a bridge between personal continuity and social engagement.

9

Conclusions and implications

REVISITING MIDLIFE AND BEYOND

Readers who have continued this far have now reached a way station in their journey through ideas and their possible consequences for mature ageing. Along the way a number of features have been observed. First, there has been a movement away from specified age-stages towards metaphors of transition, to such an extent that midlifestyles appear as fixed states, consisting of continual transitions of one sort or another. This differs from a view that transitions are points of difficulty between otherwise unproblematic life-stages. Rather, the maintenance of a believable identity has become a matter of ongoing negotiation. Both of these understandings, the modernist and the postmodern, tend to de-emphasize problematic aspects of the ageing process itself and its influence on the layering of the psyche. Second, it has become clear that the structuring of mature imagination varies markedly over personal and historical time, which can lead to conflicts associated with age being characterized differently. In some cases the question has been posed in terms of increased social potential versus restricted social possibilities. In others, personal and social possibilities appear to have increased, but include a denial of limitation and finitude. Third, the recognition of multiple possibilities for self-presentation may often be at odds with more fundamental questions of ageing. It has contributed to a particular layering of self-experience and an emphasis on both depth and surface elements, the boundary between them being negotiated through masquerade. Age has, in other words, led to the reinvention of distinctions between hidden and apparent identities. Finally, the question still remains: of what a genuine experience of mature identity is like. It is not a reworking of a previous phase of life; neither is it an invention, uprooted from personal and historical experience. Insofar as there is an answer, it may lie in spaces that facilitate a negotiated coming together of personal and intersubjective truths.

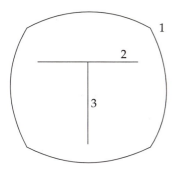

1 Social space facilitates likelihood of a particular relationship between 2 and 3
2 Surfaces for multiple statements
3 Layering of the psyche: masquerade, existential issues, active imagination, lifeforce.

Figure 9.1 A model for the mature imagination.

A MODEL FOR THE MATURE IMAGINATION

It follows from the argument above that a space in which genuine age-ing identities can emerge should contain certain recognizable qualities. It should, first and foremost, allow harmony between deeper, personal, layers of the psyche and intersubjectively agreed, social, possibilities of self-expression. This is what is meant by the merger of inner and external logics, the ability to think reflectively as well as reflexively and an atten-tion to continuity of identity as well as its immediate cohesion. Second, it should recognize the function of masque as both a protective and a con-nective performance of mature identity and allow for an element of play-fulness in this expression of self. While recognizing a new flexibility of identity that has emerged under post-Fordist, post-Eriksonian and post-stateist conditions, recognition is also needed of hidden desires in later life, which may require the performance of masquerade in order to test out new spaces that emerge. Third, these spaces must combine the facilitative qualities outlined above with an ability to sustain a containing environment. In other words, the space itself should have protective qualities that render it safe for experiments in new ways of living. In each case, a balance has to be achieved between the need for personal expression and the social and physical boundaries arising as part of the ageing process.

The model in Figure 9.1 describes, albeit in a simplified form, the key characteristics that may need to be considered in apprehending the mature imagination. Each element of the figure is fluid and reciprocal, such that a change to one would occasion changes to the other parts.

First, the opportunities for adopting different social roles and identity statements are represented by a horizontal line. This line corresponds to the surfaces presented by a postmodern understanding of identity and represents the multiplicity which is such an inviting aspect of these ideas. It adds breadth to social possibility. The elements of identity that appear along this line would, of course, be graded in terms of status and power relations; however, this is not the determining element of his or her positioning within the model. They appear as the possibilities open to any one person at any one time and correspond to that person's apprehension of the external logic of his or her immediate circumstances. These options are described along a horizontal continuum because that is how they appear to the psyche. They are not, in other words, an issue of depth. The continuum itself may include a variety of attributes, such as complexity and accessibility, which the person perceives to be salient and which influence his or her identity choice. They are the concrete manifestations of the possibilities inherent within a particular social space.

Second, a vertical line, extending downwards from the horizontal, represents the layering of the individual psyche. At surface layers, identity is represented through the medium of social masking and masquerade. These take the form of postures and stratagems adopted in order to negotiate a compromise between the social possibilities existing within the horizontal horizon and the fears and desires arising from the inner logic of the psyche. A key contemporary socio-historical manifestation of these layerings can be seen in the midlifestyles described in Chapter 5. Within such arrangements causality is fuzzy. It may not be possible to discern whether a performance depends more upon inner or outer logic. However, the adoption of masquerade may be experienced as a distinguishing feature, protecting the inner from the outer and marking a boundary between them. As has been discussed in Chapters 3 and 4, the permeability of the mask, its flexibility and the degree of choice and awareness experienced by the wearer might vary depending upon age and circumstance. Beyond layers concerning the deployment of masquerade lie core elements of the inner logic of the self. In mature adulthood, these may include some of the issues described in Chapter 6. In some respects the identity behind the mask may be the product of a self-conscious act of deception or protection. This may be the case for, example, with mature sexuality in a hostile environment. In others, apprehension of what has been hidden is more nebulous: it drifts in and out of conscious awareness, leaving a signature that is sometimes decipherable and sometimes not. Anxiety and the apprehension of finitude may form such a relationship. The active imagination would work primarily within these psychological parameters and engage in a dialogue between such existential concerns and still deeper formations, unconscious material and emanations of life force. At this depth, perception is liminal, and can be as much an awareness of connection as the perception of form and identity. In lifecourse terms, vertical layerings would concern continuity of identity, memory and the pursuit of life themes. Horizontal coherence would be more of an issue of cohesion: whether a particular identity statement 'held together' in a convincing manner within a particular social space.

The two continua described above concern the inner and outer logics of identity formations. The degree to which they come together, and in what combination, largely depends upon the nature of the social space in which they take place. A merger of these two logics, and thereby the surfacing of deeper psychological concerns, would influence the perception of how genuinely identity can be expressed. Social space occurs in the model as a circle surrounding the vertical and horizontal continua. A key quality of social space from this perspective is the degree to which it can contain reflexive and reflective awareness, as described in Chapter 7. Social spaces may be facilitative. They may, in other words, allow people to situate their thoughts and feelings and increase the possibilities for understanding the influence of internal and external logics upon the self. They may also be coercive, and lead to the suppression of thought, feeling and activity that does not fit the parameters of that particular space. If the space is hostile to the expression of mature identity, it will then give rise to a more rigid split between the apparent and the hidden and a more extensive adoption of masquerade. Social spaces are socio-historical constructs, and they contribute to the particular form that vertical layering takes and the possibilities inherent in a horizontal continuum. In this sense, the discussions of age and identity contained in Chapters 1 and 2 (psychoanalysis, ego and analytic psychology), and Chapters 7 and 8 (social policy) describe particular spaces in which the mature imagination has been shaped.

It is intended that the model described above be heuristic rather than any form of definitive statement. It simply describes one way of understanding identity which highlights the relationship between the personal and the social. It is one way, and may not necessarily be the best way, of coming to an understanding of mature adulthood. It does, however, constitute an attempt to bring together surface, depth and social circumstance without the opacity of proclaiming the primacy of one over another.

AGE AND THE STUDY OF IDENTITY

The approach to adult identity described throughout this book does lead to some, at first glance, rather peculiar implications for the theory and practice of working with age, both as a personal and as a professional project. Most of these involve the tacit age-grading that is so often a part of social institutions.

First, attention must be paid to the relative ability of spaces to contain genuine expressions of mature imagination. There is a tension between the layering of the psyche and the veracity of reports. If the space is not facilitative then all an observer, quality assessor or researcher perceives will be the contours of a masquerade. It follows that he or she will gain access to only superficial layers of meaning, leaving enduring desires and concerns untouched. This leads to a consideration of the nature of facilitative space, which, at least theoretically, has been described as one in which inner and outer logics merge. More work needs to be done, however, on an operational definition of such phenomena.

Second, social spaces are age-sensitized spaces. They contain certain assumptions about not only the relative value of priorities arising at different points in the lifecourse, but also the likelihood that these differences will be expressed. This observation suggests a need for special attention to be paid to age as an element in who speaks, makes decisions for whom and with what priorities in mind. If there are radically different logics at work at different phases of the adult lifecourse, then the apprehension of the priorities of another age-group becomes problematic. If legitimacy and power are age-stratified, it becomes important to know who in an agency decides and how far age is a factor in understanding the requirements of other groups. The age structuration of organizations, communities and other groupings now becomes an issue.

Third, awareness of the balance achieved between masquerade and deeper self-expression varies depending on age and social space. At certain phases of the adult lifecourse, where a comfortable mask has become relatively fixed, the wearer may not distinguish between masquerade and self. This may be the case even if identity is performed within a facilitative and containing space. By contrast, finding oneself in a constraining space may lead to continual tension between an emerging mature imagination and social expectation. This tension may be interpreted as resistance, pathology or sheer bloody-mindedness, the labelling of which would imply radically different courses of action for the self and for others. An appreciation of these contingencies would mean that, rather than being seen simply as a form of inauthenticity, masque should be valued as an adaptive response to inhospitable settings.

Fourth, the book is still open on the question of whether the lifecourse has its own logic. Most of the theoretical positions discussed here assume a certain series of priorities of mature identity that cannot be fully explained by recourse to social construction. For example, the ageing of the body continues regardless of lifestyle, and is fulcral to postmodern interpretations of mature adulthood; the active imagination achieves salience with advancing years and provokes a conflict with earlier life priorities; generativity is perceived as in many respects a natural reproductive aspect of human development. If it is the case that elements of ageing have a logic of their own, this deserves a certain respect, and questions therapeutic objectives aimed at the reinvention of identity based upon the immediate priorities of the here and now. It is instructive, in this context, to observe the frequency with which identity is described as a personal myth within the literature of narrative therapy. Myth implies a creation of fantasy, with little if any grounding in historical events. Perhaps we should begin to think a little more in terms of legends, which, when associations of grandiosity are cleared away, refer to the interpretation of memory and historical record. They are thereby anchored in some form of external reality.

Fifth, the unpeeling of experience from age structuration and measurement suggests that age subjectivity, cohort and chronology should be clearly distinguished both conceptually and empirically. It destabilizes the easy assumption that mature imagination can be deduced simply by working backwards from fixed categories. They contribute to the delineation of social space, but provoke a variety of associations and reactions at the personal level. Indeed, where conduct is determined by the uniformities of cohort and chronology, it is almost certain that a space has emerged in which the diversity that accompanies adult ageing has been subject to suppression.

Finally, attention to the diverse possibilities that emerge as maturity takes shape provokes its own form of reflexivity. While the role of theory and theorists has traditionally been to interpret ageing, perhaps it is also true that the interpretations they make are age-dependent. Should attention move, for example, from postmodern theories of ageing to ageing and the popularity of postmodern theory. Perhaps we should begin to think of the age of theorizing as well as the theorizing of age, as a preoccupation with reinvention, for example, reflecting the priorities of midlife Peter and Petra Pans, albeit at a particular historical juncture.

QUESTIONS FOR RESEARCH

Preliminary conclusions concerning the formulation of mature identity indicate that, in future, greater research emphasis may need to be placed on the following:

1 A recognition of the negotiated and performative nature of identities and the effects of legitimizing spaces created by policy initiatives and wider social trends. That is, greater understanding is needed of the conditions under which certain sorts of performance take place, along with examination of the personal strategies adopted by participants and their effects on the successful negotiation of helping situations.
2 It now appears that human services concerned with later-life are dealing with at least two identity dimensions: negotiations across the professional and everyday divide and those between generations, the effects of which can be expected to be cumulative and mutative. The relationships between age and position in the system have not been

fully examined to date and suggest research questions around the construction of problem areas.

3 Work on identity management and social relationships is becoming more fluid for both older people and helping professionals, and includes trends towards interdisciplinarity, partnership and stakeholding. Conceptions of identity in later life are themselves becoming more diverse, such that older people are likely to make different demands on service systems from those traditionally made. The effects on service demand and legitimacy require further investigation.

4 A study of the relationship between the intended and unintended implications of particular initiatives by an examination of their tacit as well as explicit logics. Confusions might arise, for example, between participation and responding to health and welfare need, such that participation is in itself perceived as fulfilling mature adults' requirements. It is also unclear what happens to those who do not or cannot articulate their desires within this system.

5 The emergence of multiple options and layers of identity raises the question of multiple perspective. How far do such perspectives overlap? How are gaps recognized, negotiated or legitimized? We may be moving away from problems associated with uniformity of delivery towards problems of diversity and uncertainty. These trends suggest an assessment of the degree of overlap of perception between groups and factors that contribute to effective co-working, plus an examination of gaps that emerge in policy and practice and contribute to the emergence of 'risky' spaces or 'no identity zones'.

6 There would also appear to be a need to develop research tools that can identify the phenomena highlighted by the current perspective. These include a means of operationalizing the relationship between policy and the creation of legitimizing spaces for professional–user interaction, the distinction between masquerade and more fundamental expressions of self, including the interaction between surface options and layering of identity, and the relationship between inner and outer logics.

QUESTIONS FOR PSYCHOTHERAPY

Perhaps the most obvious, yet telling, conclusion to emphasize for the talking therapies is that age is not a barrier to work with mature adults. Rather, age has become a significant factor, not only in the question of access to counselling and psychotherapy, but also as an influence on the quality of relationship that develop between client and therapist and the different levels at which such work might take place.

The implications for practice are therefore considerable. First, it is important to recognize the role of psychotherapy itself as a space which shapes social and personal possibility. In particular, it is necessary to become sensitized to the pervasive influence on child-centred theorising. This not only privileges early experience, it also casts the older adult as the villain of the piece. According to this view, your parents screw you up, whether they wish to or not. In intergenerational terms, this leaves the older client with a considerable barrier to overcome when faced with the younger therapist. If the therapeutic encounter is to become a space in which the inner world is respected, allowed free expression and protection from social prejudice, these theoretical biases must be recognized and their impact countered. Second, it has become clear that the mature imagination is itself multifaceted and that within the inner world of the older adult a number of age-specific identities may coexist. This point has a number of implications, most notably for the variety of possibilities for transference and countertransference phenomena that a therapist and client might encounter when working together. Adult age, in other words, is an important source of structuration for the human psyche. Third, the possibility of difference between the existential priorities of younger and later adulthood should be recognized as an important factor patterning the progress of therapy, the conflicts that arise and the acceptability of potential resolution. This difference introduces a fourth factor, concerning the impact of ageist environments on personal growth and development. This impact is double edged. On the one hand prejudice against mature imagination may have lead to the performance of a deeply embedded masquerade, employed to protect the self from external attack. On the other, rather than forcing personal identity into a fixed position, the diversity of identity promised under postmodern conditions may leave no place for the consideration of core existential questions that arise in midlife and beyond. The mature psyche, as it appears in therapeutic encounters, may thus be multilayered, multifaceted and confronted by dizzying yet insubstantial variety. Under such conditions, critical attention might need to be given to the relationship between the invention of personal narratives and the maintenance of continuity of identity.

QUESTIONS FOR HEALTH AND SOCIAL CARE

A significant conclusion of the current argument is that the 'modern' vision of the lifecourse, dominant in the 1950s and 1960s and influential in the shaping of contemporary health and welfare policy, has come under increasing strain as social change and technical advance have gathered pace. Three factors have contributed to this rethinking of mature identity, which will effect expectations of psychological and physical well-being. These factors include an erosion of rigid divisions between age-groups, experiment with a variety of lifestyles by older adults themselves and therapeutic and technological advances that increase bodily potential. Lifestyle choices contain a mixture of enhanced potential and avoidance of fundamental ageing processes, and present challenges some of which are familiar and some quite new. These challenges include: a concentration of age-specific populations with associated health and social needs, which in some cases exhibit an absence of intergenerational supports; the adoption of healthy lifestyles combined with the sanction of exclusion in cases of 'health failure'; and a demand for services that maintain participation and positive self-perception.

Thus, while these 'alternative' lifestyles may promote a healthy and participative old age, they may also be prone to individual cases of catastrophic collapse. This collapse is intensified by an absence of, and in some cases hostility to, intergenerational support and a climate of denial concerning legitimate dependency and age-related decrements. Where health and social needs are identified by this population they are likely to be geared towards bodily and social maintenance rather than palliative care. In many ways, lifestyle communities reproduce some of the classic aspects of institutionalization: concentrations of need, often unaddressed, but this time expressed by a vociferous and increasingly sophisticated population. They are reflected in the growth of retirement communities, seasonal migration among people for whom one residence is a second homeland and a seemingly insatiable appetite for localities previously associated with leisure, such as the seaside in British late-life. Service demand reflects a ghettoization of high-demand groups and a possible transfer of services away from chronicity and towards the problems of vocal and resource-rich elements of the ageing population.

Demands for health interventions based on lifestyle are in a reciprocal relationship with advances in medical technology. Together they mark a fundamental shift in perceptions of the ageing body, which is now seen as both a barrier to lifestyle choice and more malleable. Advances in cosmetic surgery, genetics and pharmacology, and a growing and sophisticated range of prosthetic options, have led to a decoupling of bodily, chronological and social-psychological ageing. These developments have contributed, in the popular imagination, to the possibility of reshaping the body and revising the ageing process. It is reflected in the growth of best-selling manuals that encourage the reader to maintain a midlifestyle, or abolish ageing altogether. The ageing body, in other words, need no longer be a barrier to self-enhancement. This is not simply a matter of medical progress. Something very different is happening to our cultural understanding of ageing. Ageing, in the minds of many patients, is becoming an option, even though this may simply reflect a heady mixture of public faith in medical science and an unwillingness to adapt consumer lifestyles to new circumstances.

The cultural momentum engendered by this changing relationship to the body is, arguably, familiar to helping professionals who are subject to patients' perplexity and dismay if a convincing remedy cannot be supplied for a particular complaint. There may even have been a move towards 'recreational surgery' (Hodgekin 1996); in other words, interventions that enhance beyond normative standards of performance and repair. Concepts of normality have a history of misuse, in the service of a prejudicial denial of services to older adults. However, trends identified above might also predict greater sensitivity to distinctions based on the ethics of medical interventions to enhance performance. This debate approximates that surrounding the recreational use of steroids and is suggestive of demands over and above the palliative and cure, to enhancement beyond what the body and mind are ordinarily capable of. In terms of health and social care, we would no longer be guided by late-life as 'downhill all the way', but be entering new territory in terms of how older people might be living, and their expectations. The shaping of mature identity in ways that largely avoid or deny questions of ageing would indicate the need for counselling and educational services that can offer lifecourse advice. Issues, for example, the deployment of masquerade and existential questions that are often left unaddressed might then be subject to negotiation. This service would extend to the mediation of intergenerational relationships, especially where these have become troubled.

Trends in demography, lifestyle and health technology, then, may significantly influence future demand for health-related services in later life. Specifically, trends point to a growth in demand for therapies of bodily maintenance and enhancement, in addition to the more traditional care of chronic conditions. The populations generating these demands may differ depending on geography and socio-economic status, with vocal and affluent concentrations contrasted with patients who are both socially marginalized and geographically dispersed. Groups generating novel demands would have many positive attributes in terms of healthy lifestyle and have, by degrees, bought the message of health promotion. However, rather than reducing service requirements, lifestyle changes may have simply changed the nature of demands being made. These trends pose significant challenges to the contemporary orthodoxies of health and social care, which include re-examining notions of normality in late-life development, the impact of lifestyle change on demand for services and the strategic impact of concentrated age-specific groupings. Developments are complicated by a widespread denial of existential questions and performative aspects of identity during the mature lifecourse. A fuller understanding of the fears and desires that drive contemporary patterns requires a more sophisticated apprehension of the mature imagination, to which this book is a contribution.

References

Abraham, K. (1919) The applicability of psychoanalytic treatment to patients of an advanced age. In *Selected Papers on Psychoanalysis*. London: Hogarth.

Alexander, B., Rubenstein, R., Goodman, M. and Loborsky, M. (1992) Generativity in cultural context, *Ageing and Society*, 11, 417–42.

Amin, K. and Patel, N. (1998) *Growing Old Far from Home*. London: Runnymede.

Andrews, M. (1991) *Lifetimes of Commitment*. Cambridge: Cambridge University Press.

Arber, S. and Ginn, J. (1995) *Connecting Gender and Ageing*. Buckingham: Open University Press.

Atchley, R. (1989) A continuity theory of normal aging, *The Gerontologist*, 29, 183–90.

Atchley, R. (1991) The influence of aging or frailty on perceptions and expressions of the self. In J. Birren (ed.) *The Concept and Measurement of Quality of Life in the Frail Elderly*. New York: Academic Press.

Atkinson, K. (1996) The community of strangers: supervision and the new right, *Health and Social Care in the Community*, 4(2), 122–5.

Austin, C. and O'Connor, K. (1989) Case management, components and program contexts. In M. Peterson and D. White (eds) *Health Care of the Elderly*. New York: Sage.

Baars, J. and Thomese, F. (1994) Communes for elderly people, *Journal of Aging Studies*, 8(4), 341–56.

Baddeley, S. (1995) Internal polity, *Human Relations*, 48(9), 1073–103.

Baltes, M. and Carstensen, L. (1996) The process of successful ageing, *Ageing and Society*, 16, 397–422.

Banks, J. (1996) The sad but instructive case of Virginia Woolf, *Journal of Aging and Identity*, 1(1), 23–35.

Baudrillard, J. (1990) *Fatal Strategies*. New York: Semiotexte.

Baudrillard, J. (1993) *Symbolic Exchange and Death*. London: Sage.

Bauman, Z. (1995) *Life in Fragments: Essays in Postmodern Morality*. Oxford: Blackwell.

Bauman, Z. (1997) *Postmodernity and Its Discontents*. Cambridge: Polity Press.

Bauman, Z. (1998) What prospects of morality in times of uncertainty? *Theory, Culture and Society*, 15(1), 11–22.

Baumhover, L. and Beall, S. (1996) *Abuse, Neglect and Exploitation of Older Persons*. London: Jessica Kingsley.

Beckingham, A. (1997) Interdisciplinary health care teamwork in the care of the elderly, *Bold*, 7(2), 17–23.

Berger, P. and Luckman, T. (1971) *The Social Construction of Reality*. London: Allen Lane.

Berman, M. (1982) *All that Is Solid Melts into Air*. London: Verso.

Bernard, M. and Meade, K. (1993) *Women Come of Age*. London: Edward Arnold.

Beveridge, W. (1942) *Report on Social Assistance*, Cmd 6404. London: HMSO.

Biggs, S. (1989) Professional helpers and resistances to work with older people, *Ageing and Society*, 9(1), 43–60.

Biggs, S. (1990a) Consumers, case management and inspection, *Critical Social Policy*, 30, 23–38.

Biggs, S. (1990b) Ageism and confronting ageing, *Journal of Social Work Practice*, 4(2), 43–65.

Biggs, S. (1991) Community care, case management and the psychodynamic perspective, *Journal of Social Work Practice*, 5(1), 71–81.

Biggs, S. (1993a) *Understanding Ageing*. Buckingham: Open University Press.

Biggs, S. (1993b) User participation and interprofessional collaboration in community care, *Journal of Interprofessional Care*, 7(2), 151–9.

Biggs, S. (1994) Failed individualism in community care: an example from elder abuse, *Journal of Social Work Practice*, 8(2), 137–51.

Biggs, S. (1996) Elder abuse and the policing of community care, *Generations Review*, 6(2), 2–4.

Biggs, S. (1997a) Interprofessional collaboration: problems and prospects. In J. Øvretveit, P. Mathias and T. Thompson (eds) *Interprofessional Working for Health and Social Care*. London: Macmillan.

Biggs, S. (1997b) User voice, interprofessionalism and postmodernity, *Journal of Interprofessional Care*, 11(2), 195–203.

Biggs, S. (1997c) Choosing not to be old? Masks, bodies and identity management in later life, *Ageing and Society*, 17(5), 533–53.

Biggs, S. (1998) Mature imaginations: ageing and the psychodynamic tradition, *Ageing and Society*, 18, 1–19.

Biggs, S., Kingston, P., Bernard, M. and Nettleton, H. (1998) Health, identity and age-specific housing. Paper presented to European Conference of Social Gerontology, Helsinki.

Biggs, S., Phillipson, C. and Kingston, P. (1995) *Elder Abuse in Perspective*. Buckingham: Open University Press.

Billig, M. (1997) Freud and Dora, *Theory, Culture and Society*, 14(3), 45–52.

Bion, W. (1961) *Experiences in Groups*. London: Tavistock.

Blair, T. (1996) *New Britain: My Vision of a New Country*. London: Fourth Estate.

Blakemore, K. (1998) Migration and lifestories. In K. Amin and N. Patel (eds) *Growing Old Far from Home*. London: Runnymede.

Boateng, P. (1997) *Seminar on the Abuse of Vulnerable Adults*. London: Department of Health.

Bollas, C. (1989) *Forces of Destiny*. London: Free Association Books.

Bond, J. (1992) The politics of caregiving: the professionalisation of informal care, *Ageing and Society*, 12, 5–21.

Bott-Spillius, E. (1988) *Melanie Klein Today, Volume 1: Mainly Theory*. London: Routledge.

Brammer, A. (1994) The registered homes act; safeguarding the elderly? *Journal of Social Welfare and Family Law*, 16(4), 423.

Brammer, A. and Biggs, S. (1998) Defining elder abuse, *Journal of Social Welfare and Family Law*, 20(3), 285–304.

Brecher, E. (1993) *Love, Sex and Aging: a Consumer Union Report*. Boston: Little Brown.

Brennan, T. (1997) The two forms of consciousness, *Theory, Culture and Society*, 14(4), 88–96.

Breuer, J. and Freud, S. (1895) *Studies on Hysteria*. Harmondsworth: Penguin.

Brim, O. (1974) *Selected Theories of the Male Midlife Crisis*. New Orleans: APA.

Brooke, R. (1991) *Jung and Phenomenology*. London: Routledge.

Burman, E. (1996) False memories, true hopes and the angelic: revenge of the postmodern in therapy, *New Formations*, 30, 122–34.

Buss, A. (1979) Dialectics, history and development. In P. Baltes and O. Brim (eds) *Lifespan Development and Behaviour, Volume 2*. New York: Academic Press.

Butler, J. (1996) Gender as performance. In P. A. Osbourne (ed.) *Critical Sense*. London: Routledge.

Butler, R. (1963) The life review an interpretation of reminiscence in the aged, *Psychiatry*, 26, 65–76.

Butler, R. (1975) *Why Survive? Being Old in America*. San Francisco: Harper and Row.

Butler, R. (1987) Agism. In *The Encyclopaedia of Aging*. New York: Springer.

Callahan, J. and Lansbery, S. (1997) Can we tap the power of NORCs? *Perspectives on Aging*, 26(1), 13–20.

Camara, V. (1997) Interdisciplinary elderly care: report of an experience, *Bold*, 7(2), 18–21.

Caputo, R. (1988) *Management and Information Systems in Human Services*. New York: Haworth.

Carlin, J. (1996) The loneliness of the long distance stunner, *Independent*, 19 May.

Castoriades, C. (1997) The crisis of the identification process, *Thesis Eleven*, 49, 45–68.

Cheston, R. (1996) Stories and metaphors, talking about the past in a psychotherapy group for people with dementia, *Ageing and Society*, 16, 579–602.

Chinen, A. (1989) *In the Ever-after*. Wilmette, IL: Chiron.

Chodorow, J. (1997) *Jung on Active Imagination*. London: Routledge.

Chopra, D. (1993) *Ageless Body, Timeless Mind: a Practical Alternative to Growing Old*. New York: Rider Books.

Cohler, B. (1993) Aging, morale and meaning. In T. Cole (ed.) *Voices and Visions of Aging*. New York: Springer.

Coleman, P. (1986) *Ageing and Reminiscence Processes*. Chichester: Wiley.

Coleman, P. (1996) Identity management in later life. In R. Woods (ed.) *Handbook of the Clinical Psychology of Ageing*. Chichester: Wiley.

Colthart, N. (1991) the analysis of an elderly patient, *International Journal of Psychoanalysis*, 72(2), 209–19.

Comley, M. (1998) Counselling and therapy with older refugees, *Journal of Social Work Practice*, 12(2), 141–53.

Conrad, C. (1992) Old age in a modern and postmodern world. In R. Cole, D. van Tassel and R. Kastenbaum (eds) *Handbook of the Humanities and Aging*. New York: Springer.

Conway, M. (1990) *Autobiographical Memory*. Buckingham: Open University Press.

Cooper, A. (1996) Psychoanalysis and the politics of organisational theory, *Journal of Social Work Practice*, 10(2), 137–46.

Corrigan, P. and Leonard, P. (1981) *Social Work Practice under Capitalism*. London: Macmillan.

Coupland, J., Coupland, N. and Grainger, K. (1991) Intergenerational discourse: contextual versions of ageing and elderliness, *Ageing and Society*, 11, 189–208.

Crews, F. (1997) *The Memory Wars: Freud's Legacy in Dispute*. London: Granata.

Croft, S. and Beresford, P. (1992) The politics of participation, *Critical Social Policy*, 35, 20–44.

Crook, S., Pakulski, J. and Waters, M. (1992) *Postmodernization*. London: Sage.

Cumming, E. and Henry, W. (1961) *Growing Old*. New York: Basic Books.

Cutler, N. (1997) Financial gerontology and the middle-ageing of the world, *Generations Review*, 7(2), 4–6.

Dante, A. (1307) *The Divine Comedy*, trans. D. Sayers, 1949. Harmondsworth: Penguin.

Dartington, T. (1986) *The Limits of Altruism*. London: Kings Fund.

Davis, H. (1996) Psychodynamics and empowerment in community mental health, *Journal of Social Work Practice*, 10(2), 157–62.

Dean, H. and Taylor-Gooby, P. (1992) *Dependency Culture*. London: Harvester Wheatsheaf.

de Beauvoir, S. (1970) *Old Age*. Harmondsworth: Penguin.

Decalmer, P. and Glendenning, F. (1993) *The Mistreatment of Elderly People*. London: Sage.

Department of Health (1991) *Community Care in the Next Decade and Beyond*. London: HMSO.

Dittman-Kohli, F. (1991) The construction of meaning in old age, *Ageing and Society*, 10, 279–94.

Eastman, M. (1984) *Old Age Abuse*. Mitcham: Age Concern.

Elkins, D., Hedstrom, L., Hughes, L., Leaf, J. and Saunders, J. (1988) Towards a humanistic, phenomenological spirituality, *Journal of Humanistic Psychology*, 28, 5–18.

Ellman, R. (1949) *Yeats: the Man and the Masks*. London: Macmillan.

Erikson, E. (1950) *Childhood and Society*. New York: Norton.

Erikson, E. (1959) *Identity and the Lifecycle*. New York: Norton.

Erikson, E. (1963) *Childhood and Society*, rev. edn. New York: Norton.

Erikson, E. (1982) *The Life Cycle Completed*. New York: Norton.

Erikson, E., Erikson, J. and Kivnick, H. (1986) *Vital Involvement in Old Age*. New York: Norton.

Estes, C. (1979) *The Aging Enterprise*. San Francisco: Jossey-Bass.

Estes, C., Swan, J. and associates (1993) *The Long Term Care Crisis: Elders Trapped in the No Care Zone*. Newbury Park, CA: Sage.

Etzioni, A. (1997) *The Golden Rule: Community and Morality in a Democratic Society*. New York: Profile Books.

Evers, H., Cameron, E. and Badger, F. (1994) Interprofessional work with old and disabled people. In A. Leathard (ed.) *Going Interprofessional: Working Together for Health and Welfare*. London: Routledge.

Fairhurst, E. (1997) Recalling life: analytical issues in the use of 'memories'. In A. Jamieson, S. Harper and C. Victor (eds) *Critical Approaches to Ageing and Later Life*. Buckingham: Open University Press.

Falk, P. (1995) Written in the flesh, *Body and Society*, 1(1), 95–105.

Farrell, M. (1975) Unpublished paper, cited in Guttman (1975).

Featherstone, M. (1983) Consumer culture: an introduction, *Theory, Culture and Society*, 1(3), 1–8.

Featherstone, M. (1991) *Consumer Culture and Postmodernism*. London: Sage.

Featherstone, M. and Hepworth, M. (1982) Ageing and inequality: consumer culture and the new middle age. In D. Robbins (ed.) *Rethinking Inequality*. London: Gower.

Featherstone, M. and Hepworth, M. (1983) The midlifestyle of 'George and Lynne', *Theory, Culture and Society*, 1(3), 85–92.

Featherstone, M. and Hepworth, M. (1989) Ageing and old age: reflections on the postmodern lifecourse. In B. Bytheway (ed.) *Becoming and Being Old*. London: Sage.

Featherstone, M. and Hepworth, M. (1990) Images of ageing. In J. Bond and P. Coleman (eds) *Ageing in Society*. London: Sage.

Featherstone, M. and Hepworth, M. (1991) The mask of ageing and the postmodern lifecourse. In M. Featherstone, M. Hepworth and B. S. Turner (eds) *The Body, Social Process and Cultural Theory*. London: Sage.

Featherstone, M. and Hepworth, M. (1995) Images of positive ageing. In M. Featherstone and A. Wernick (eds) *Images of Ageing*. London: Routledge.

Featherstone, M. and Wernick, A. (eds) (1995) *Images of Ageing*. London: Routledge.

Feinstein, D. (1997) Personal mythology and psychotherapy, *American Journal of Orthopsychiatry*, 67(4), 508–22.

Finch, J. (1995) Responsibilities, obligations and commitments. In I. Allen and E. Perkins (eds) *The Future of Family Care for Older People*. London: HMSO.

Forbes, J. and Sashidharan, S. (1997) User involvement in services: incorporation of challenge? *British Journal of Social Work*, 27(4), 481–99.

Fordham, F. (1956) *An Introduction to Jung's Psychology*. Harmondsworth: Penguin.

Foucault, M. (1977) *Discipline and Punish*. New York: Sheridan.

Foucault, M. (1979) *History of Sexuality, Volume 1*. Harmondsworth: Penguin.

Frankl, V. (1955) *The Doctor and the Soul*. Harmondsworth: Penguin.

Frankl, V. (1969) *Psychotherapy and Existentialism*. Harmondsworth: Penguin.

Freire, P. (1972) *Pedagogy of the Oppressed*. Harmondsworth: Penguin.

Freud, S. (1897) *Sexual Aetiology of the Neuroses. Collected Works, 1*. London: Hogarth.

Freud, S. (1901) *The Psychopathology of Everyday Life. Collected Works, 6*. London: Hogarth.

Freud, S. (1905) *On Psychotherapy. Collected Works, 7*. London: Hogarth.

Freud, S. (1912) *Types of Onset of the Neuroses. Collected Works, 12*. London: Hogarth.

Freud, S. (1920) *Beyond the Pleasure Principle. Collected Works, 18*. London: Hogarth.

Freud, S. (1930) *Civilization and Its Discontents. Collected Works, 21*. London: Hogarth.

Fromm, E. (1956) *The Sane Society*. London: Routledge.

Frosh, S. (1989) Melting into air: psychoanalysis and social experience. *Free Associations*, 16, 7–30.

Frosh, S. (1991) *Identity Crisis: Modernity, Psychoanalysis and the Self.* London: Macmillan.

Gellhorn, L. (1997) *Independent*, 14 January.

Gergen, K. (1991) *The Saturated Self: Dilemmas of Identity in Contemporary Life.* New York: Basic Books.

Gibson, F. (1997) Political violence and coping in Northern Ireland. In L. Hunt, M. Marshall and C. Rawlings (eds) *Past Trauma in Late Life.* London: Jessica Kingsley.

Giddens, A. (1991) *Modernity and Self-identity.* Cambridge: Polity Press.

Giles, H. and Coupland, N. (1991) *Language, Contexts and Consequences.* Buckingham: Open University Press.

Gilleard, C. (1996) Consumption and identity in later life, *Ageing and Society*, 16, 489–98.

Goffman, E. (1960) *Asylums.* Harmondsworth: Penguin.

Goffman, E. (1961) *The Presentation of Self in Everyday Life.* Harmondsworth: Penguin.

Goffman, E. (1963) *Stigma.* Harmondsworth: Penguin.

Goffman, E. (1967) *Interaction Ritual.* Harmondsworth: Penguin.

Greer, G. (1991) *The Change: Women Ageing and the Menopause.* Harmondsworth: Penguin.

Grotjahn, M. (1955) Analytic psychotherapy with the elderly. *Psychoanalytic Review*, 42, 419–27.

Gubrium, J. (1993) *Speaking of Life: Horizons of Meaning for Nursing Home Residents.* New York: Walther de Gruyter.

Gubrium, J. and Wallace, J. (1990) Who theorises age? *Ageing and Society*, 10, 131–49.

Guttman, D. (1975) Individual adaptation in the middle years, *Boston Society for Gerontologic Psychiatry*, 5(31), 41–59.

Guttman, D. (1987) *Reclaimed Powers.* London: Hutchinson.

Hallett, C. and Birchall, E. (1992) *Coordination and Child Protection.* London: HMSO.

Haraway, D. (1991) *Simians, Cyborgs and Women.* London: Free Association Books.

Hassan, J. (1997) From victim to survivor: the possibility of healing in ageing survivors of the Nazi Holocaust. In L. Hunt, M. Marshall and C. Rawlings (eds) *Past Trauma in Late Life.* London: Jessica Kingsley.

Healey, S. (1994) Growing to be an old woman. In E. Stoller and R. Gibson (eds) *Worlds of Difference: Inequality in the Aging Experience.* Thousand Oaks, CA: Pine Forge Press.

Heidegger, M. (1926) *Being and Time.* London: Harper and Row.

Hepworth, M. (1991) Positive ageing and the mask of age, *Journal of Educational Gerontology*, 6(2), 93–101.

Higgs, P. (1995) Citizenship and old age: the end of the road? *Ageing and Society*, 15, 535–51.

Hildebrand, P. (1982) Psychotherapy with older patients, *British Journal of Medical Psychology*, 55, 19–28.

Hildebrand, P. (1986) Dynamic psychotherapy with the elderly. In I. Hanley and M. Gilhooly, M. (eds) *Psychological Therapies for the Elderly.* London: Croom Helm.

Hillman, J. (1970) *The Myth of Analysis*. Evanston, IL: Northwestern University Press.

Hinshelwood, R. (1996) The social relocation of personal identity, *Philosophy, Psychiatry and Psychology*, 2(3), 185–204.

Hobman, D. (1990) A bad business. In *Age: the Unrecognised Discrimination*. London: Age Concern.

Hodgekin, P. (1996) Medicine, postmodernism and the end of certainty, *British Medical Journal*, 313, 1568–9.

Holland, P. (1996) I've just seen a hole in the reality barrier. In H. Pilcher (ed.) *Thatcher's Children*. London: Falmer Press.

Hollender, M. (1952) Individualising the aged, *Social Casework*, 33, 337–42.

Homans, P. (1995) *Jung in Context*. Chicago: University of Chicago Press.

Hopcke, R. (1995) *Persona*. Boston: Shambhala.

Horney, K. (1955) *Self-analysis*. London: Routledge.

Howe, D. (1994) Modernity, postmodernity and social work, *British Journal of Social Work*, 24(5), 513–32.

Hughes, B. (1995) *Older People and Community Care*. Buckingham: Open University Press.

Hunt, L., Marshall, M. and Rowlings, C. (1997) *Past Trauma in Late Life*. London: Jessica Kingsley.

Ingrisch, D. (1995) Conformity and resistance as women age. In S. Arber and J. Ginn (eds) *Connecting Gender and Ageing*. Buckingham: Open University Press.

Isenberg, S. (1992) Aging in Judaism. In T. Cole, D. van Tassel and R. Kastenbaum (eds) *Handbook of the Humanities and Aging*. New York: Springer.

Itzin, C. (1986) Ageism awareness and training. In C. Phillipson, M. Bernard and P. Strang (eds) *Dependency and Interdependency in Old Age*. London: Croom Helm.

Jacobs, M. (1986) *The Presenting Past*. Buckingham: Open University Press.

Jacobson, H. (1998) *The Guardian*, 5 March.

Jameson, F. (1984) Postmodernism, or the cultural logic of late capitalism, *New Left Review*, 146, 53–92.

Jaques, E. (1955) Social systems as a defence against persecutory and depressive anxiety. In M. Klein and P. Heiman (eds) *New Directions in Psychoanalysis*. London: Tavistock.

Jaques, E. (1965) Death and the midlife crisis, *International Journal of Psychoanalysis*, 46(4), 507–14.

Jaques, E. (1995) Why the psychoanalytical approach to understanding organisations is dysfunctional, *Human Relations*, 48, 343–50.

Jordan, B. (1996) *A Theory of Poverty and Social Exclusion*. Cambridge: Polity Press.

Jung, C. (1916) *The Transcendent Function*. London: Routledge and Kegan Paul.

Jung, C. (1921) *Psychological Types*. Princeton, NJ: Princeton University Press.

Jung, C. (1931) *The Aims of Psychotherapy*. London: Routledge and Kegan Paul.

Jung, C. (1933a) *A Study in the Process of Individuation*. Princeton, NJ: Princeton University Press.

Jung, C. (1933b) *Modern Man in Search of a Soul*. London: Routledge.

Jung, C. (1935) *The Tavistock Lectures*. Princeton, NJ: Princeton University Press.

Jung, C. (1961) *Memories, Dreams, Reflections*. London: Routledge.

Jung, C. G. (1967a) *Collected Works, Volume 4*. London: Routledge.

Jung, C. G. (1967b) *Collected Works, Volume 7*. London: Routledge.

Jung, C. G. (1967c) *Collected Works, Volume 8.* London: Routledge.

Jung, C. G. (1967d) *Collected Works, Volume 9.* London: Routledge.

Jung, C. G. (1967e) *Collected Works, Volume 16.* London: Routledge.

Kaminsky, M. (1993) Definitional ceremonies: depoliticizing and reenchanting the culture of age. In T. Cole (ed.) *Voices and Visions of Aging.* New York: Springer.

Kanter, J. (1988) Clinical issues in the case management relationship. In M. Harris and L. Bacherach (eds) *Clinical Case Management.* New York: Jossey-Bass.

Kastenbaum, R. (1992) The creative process: a lifespan approach. In T. Cole, D. van Tassel and R. Kastenbaum (eds) *Handbook of the Humanities and Aging.* New York: Springer.

Kastenbaum, R. (1993) Encrusted elders: Arizona and the political spirit of post-modern aging. In T. Cole (ed.) *Voices and Visions of Aging.* New York: Springer.

Katz, S. (1996) *Disciplining Old Age.* Charlottesville, VA: University Press of Virginia.

Kaye, R. (1993) Sexuality in the later years, *Ageing and Society,* 13, 415–26.

Khaleelee, O. and Miller, E. (1985) Beyond the small group: society as an intelligible field of study. In M. Pines and W. Bion (eds) *Group Psychotherapy.* London: Routledge.

King, N. (1996) Autobiography as cultural memory, *New Formations,* 30, 50–62.

King, P. (1974) Notes on the psychoanalysis of older patients, *Journal of Analytical Psychology,* 19, 22–37.

King, P. (1980) The lifecycle as indicated by the nature of the transference in the psychoanalysis of the middle-aged and elderly, *International Journal of Psycho-analysis,* 61, 153–60.

Kingston, P. and Penhale, B. (1995) *Family Violence and the Caring Professions.* London: Macmillan.

Kitwood, T. (1997) *Dementia Reconsidered.* Buckingham: Open University Press.

Kivnick, H. (1988) Grandparenthood, life-review and psychosocial development, *Journal of Gerontological Social Work,* 12(3/4), 63–82.

Kivnick, H. (1993) Everyday mental health. In M. Symer (ed.) *Mental Health and Aging.* New York: Springer.

Kleinberg, J. (1995) Group treatment of adults in midlife, *International Journal of Group Psychotherapy,* 45(2), 207–22.

Knight, B. (1986) *Psychotherapy with Older Adults.* Beverley Hills, CA: Sage.

Knight, B. (1996) Psychodynamic therapy with older adults. In R. Woods (ed.) *Handbook of the Clinical Psychology of Ageing.* Chichester: Wiley.

Kondratowitz, H-J. (1998) A short history of social gerontology in Europe. Paper presented to European Behavioural and Social Science Research Section of The European Congress of Gerontology Symposium, Helsinki.

Kotre, J. (1984) *Outliving the Self: Generativity and the Interpretation of Lives.* Baltimore: Johns Hopkins University Press.

Krippner, S. and Winkler, M. (1995) Postmodernity and consciousness studies, *Journal of Mind and Behavior,* 16(3), 255–80.

Kuhn, M. (1977) *On Aging.* Philadelphia: Westminster.

Kumar, K. (1995) *From Post-industrial to Post-modern Society.* Oxford: Blackwell.

Lachman, M. (1986) Locus of control in aging research, *Psychology and Aging,* 1, 34–40.

Lambley, P. (1995) *The Middle-aged Rebel.* Shaftesbury: Element.

Latimer, J. (1997) The dark at the bottom of the stairs: performance and participation of hospitalised older people, *Medical Anthropology Quarterly*, 15(2), 31.

Latimer, J. (1998) Review of retirement communities. Internal paper, Keele Centre for Social Gerontology.

Lawrence, G. (1977) Management development: some ideals images and realities. In A. Coleman and M. Geller (eds) *Group Relations Reader 2*. Washington, DC: Rice Institute.

Lawrence, G. (1979) *Exploring Individual and Organizational Boundaries*. Chichester: Wiley.

Lawrence, G. (1995) Social dreaming as a tool for action research. Paper presented to the ISPSO Conference, London.

Laws, G. (1995) Embodiment and emplacement; identities, representation and landscape in Sun City retirement communities, *International Journal of Aging and Human Development*, 40(4), 253–80.

Lee, R. (1998) The tao of exchange: ideology and cosmology in Baudrillard's fatalism, *Thesis Eleven*, 52, 53–68.

Le Grand, J. and Bartlett, W. (1993) *Quasi-markets and Social Policy*. London: Macmillan.

Leonard, P. (1997) *Postmodern Welfare*. London: Sage.

Litvinoff, S. (1997) *Independent on Sunday*, 1 June.

Locke, J. (1690) *An Essay Concerning Human Understanding*. London: Fontana.

Lord Chancellor's Department (1997) *Who Decides? Making Decisions on Behalf of Mentally Incapacitated Adults*, Cm 3803. London: HMSO.

Lowe, R. (1994) Lessons from the past: the rise and fall of the classic welfare state in Britain. In A. Oakley and S. Williams (eds) *The Politics of the Welfare State*. London: UCL Press.

Lury, C. (1996) *Consumer Culture*. Cambridge: Polity Press.

Lynch, T. (1997) *The Undertaking*. London: Jonathan Cape.

Lynott, R. and Lynott, P. (1996) Tracing the course of theoretical development in the sociology of aging, *The Gerontologist*, 36(6), 749–60.

McAdams, D. (1985) *Power, Intimacy and the Lifestory*. Homewood, IL: Dorsey.

McAdams, D. (1993) *The Stories We Live By*. New York: Morrow.

McAdams, D. (1997) The case for unity in the (post) modern self. In R. Ashmore and L. Jussim (eds) *Self and Identity*. New York: Oxford University Press.

McFadden, S. (1996) Religion, spirituality and aging. In J. Birren and K. Schaie (eds) *Handbook of the Psychology of Aging*. New York: Academic Press.

McGuire, W. (ed.) (1991) *The Freud/Jung Letters*. Harmondsworth: Penguin.

McLeod, J. (1996) The emerging narrative approach to counselling and psychotherapy, *British Journal of Guidance and Counselling*, 24(2), 173–84.

MacPherson, S. (1997) Social exclusion, *Journal of Social Policy*, 26(4), 533–42.

Maquarrie, J. (1973) *Existentialism*. Harmondsworth: Penguin.

Marcia, J. (1966) Development and variation of ego-identity status, *Journal of Personality and Social Psychology*, 3, 551–8.

Marcoen, A. (1994) Spirituality and personal well-being in old age, *Ageing and Society*, 14(4), 521–36.

Marcuse, E. (1964) *One Dimensional Man*. London: Paladin.

Markus, H. and Nurius, P. (1986) Possible selves, *American Psychologist*, 41, 954–69.

Marshall, T. (1997) Infected and affected: HIV, AIDS and the older adult, *Generations Review*, 7(4), 9–12.

Marx, K. and Engels, F. (1888) *The Communist Manifesto*. Harmondsworth: Penguin (1967 edn).

Masters, W. and Johnson, V. (1970) *Human Sexual Inadequacy*. Boston: Little Brown.

Matthews, S. (1979) *The Social World of Older Women*. Beverley Hills, CA: Sage.

Mattinson, J. and Sinclair, I. (1979) *Mate and Stalemate*. Oxford: Blackwell.

Means, R. and Smith, R. (1994) *Community Care: Policy and Practice*. London: Macmillan.

Menzies, I. (1970) *The Functioning of Social Systems as a Defence against Anxiety*. London: Tavistock.

Middelcoop, P. (1985) *The Wise Old Man*. Boston: Shambhala.

Miles, J. (1994) Slow progress: why a political framework is necessary for the evaluation of pensioners campaigns, *Generations Review*, 4(1), 4–6.

Miller, E. (1993) *From Dependency to Autonomy*. London: Free Association Books.

Miller, E. and Gwynne, G. (1972) *A Life Apart*. London: Tavistock.

Miller, E. and Rice, A. (1967) *Systems of Organisation*. London: Tavistock.

Mills, M. (1997) Narrative identity and dementia, *Ageing and Society*, 17, 673–98.

Minkler, M. (1996) Critical perspective on ageing; new challenges for gerontology, *Ageing and Society*, 16(4), 467–87.

Minkler, M. and Estes, C. (1998) *Critical Gerontology*. New York: Baywood.

Minkler, M. and Robertson, A. (1991) The ideology of age-race wars, *Ageing and Society*, 11, 1–22.

Mitchell, L. and Coats, M. (1997) The functional map of health and welfare. In J. Øvretveit, P. Mathias and T. Thompson (eds) *Interprofessional Working for Health and Social Care*. London: Macmillan.

Mongardini, C. (1992) The ideology of postmodernity, *Theory, Culture and Society*, 9(2), 55–66.

Moody, H. (1986) The meaning of life and the meaning of old age. In T. Cole and S. Gaddow (eds) *What Does It Mean to Grow Old?* Durham, NC: Duke University Press.

Moody, H. (1988) Twenty five years of life-review, *Journal of Gerontological Social Work*, 12(3/4), 7–24.

Morris, J. (1991) *Pride against Prejudice*. London: The Women's Press.

Morris, J. (1992) Us and them? Feminist research, community care and disability, *Critical Social Policy*, 33, 22–39.

Moxley, D. (1989) *The Practice of Case Management*. Beverley Hills, CA: Sage.

Mullins, L. and Tucker, R. (1988) *Snowbirds in the Sunbelt*. Orlando, FL: IECG, University of South Florida.

Mulvey, L. (1991) A phantasmagoria of the female body: the work of Cindy Sherman, *New Left Review*, 188, 136–50.

Munro, R. (1996) The consumption view of self: extension, exchange and identity. In S. Edgell, K. Hetherington and A. Warde (eds) *Consumption Matters*. Oxford: Blackwell.

Munro, R. (1998) Belonging on the move: market rhetoric and the future as obligatory passage, *Sociological Review*, 46(2), 208–21.

Myers, F. and MacDonald, C. (1996) Power to the people? Involving users and carers in needs assessments and care planning – views from the practitioner, *Health and Social Care in the Community*, 4(2), 86–95.

Nathan, J. (1994) The psychic organisation of community care: a Kleinian perspective, *Journal of Social Work Practice*, 8(2), 113–22.

Nava, M. (1992) *Changing Cultures: Feminism, Youth and Consumerism*. London: Sage.

Neugarten, B. (ed.) (1968) *Middle Age and Aging*. Chicago: University of Chicago Press.

Neugarten, B. and Guttman, D. (1968) Age-sex roles and personality in middle age. In B. Neugarten (ed.) *Middle Age and Aging*. Chicago: University of Chicago Press.

Nocon, A. (1994) *Collaboration in Community Care in the 1990s*. Sunderland: Business Education Publishers.

Obholzer, A. (1993) Institutional forces, *Therapeutic Communities*, 14(4), 18–27.

Obholzer, A. and Roberts, V. (eds) (1994) *The Unconscious at Work*. London: Routledge.

O'Leary, B. (1996) *Counseling Older Adults*. London: Chapman and Hall.

Oliver, M. (1990) *The Politics of Disablement*. London: Macmillan.

O'Malley, T., Segal, H. and Perez, R. (1979) *Elder Abuse*. Boston: Legal Research and Services to the Elderly.

Øvretveit, J. (1993) *Coordinating Community Care*. Buckingham: Open University Press.

Øvretveit, J. (1997) How patient power and client participation affects relations between professionals. In J. Øvretveit, P. Mathias and T. Thompson (eds) *Interprofessional Working for Health and Social Care*. London: Macmillan.

Øvretveit, J., Mathias, P. and Thompson, T. (eds) (1997) *Interprofessional Working for Health and Social Care*. London: Macmillan.

Pahl, R. and Spencer, L. (1998) The politics of friendship, *Renewal*, 5(3/4), 100–7.

Parker, I. (1996) Postmodernism and its discontents: therapeutic discourse, *British Journal of Psychotherapy*, 12(4), 447–60.

Patel, N. (1990) *A 'Race' against Time*. London: Runnymede.

Peace, S., Kellaher, L. and Willcocks, D. (1997) *Re-evaluating Residential Care*. Buckingham: Open University Press.

Peeters, J. and Woldringh, N. (1988) *Groepswonen van Ouderen*. Nijmegen: ITS.

Penna, S. and O'Brien, M. (1996) Postmodernism and social policy, *Journal of Social Policy*, 25(1), 39–62.

Phillipson, C. (1982) *Capitalism and the Construction of Old Age*. London: Macmillan.

Phillipson, C. (1997) Social relationships in later life: a review of the research literature, *International Journal of Geriatric Psychiatry*, 12, 505–12.

Phillipson, C. (1998) *Reconstructing Old Age*. London: Sage.

Phillipson, C. and Biggs. S. (1998) Modernity and identity: themes and perspectives in the study of older adults, *Aging and Identity*, 3(1), 11–23.

Phillipson, C. and Strang, P. (1986) *Training and Education for an Ageing Society*. Keele: Keele University Press.

Phillipson, C. and Walker, A. (1986) *Social Policy and Old Age*. London: Sage.

Pillemer, K. and Wolf, R. (1986) *Elder Abuse: Conflict in the Family*. Boston: Auburn House.

Pincus, L. and Dare, C. (1978) *Secrets in the Family*. London: Faber.

Podnieks, E. (1992) National survey on abuse of the elderly in Canada, *Journal of Elder Abuse and Neglect*, 4, 5–58.

Pointon, S. (1997) Myths and negative attitudes about sexuality in older people, *Generations Review*, 7(4), 6–8.

Porter, S. (1997) The patient and power: sociological perspectives on the consequences of holistic care, *Health and Social Care in the Community*, 5(1), 17–21.

Post, S. (1992) Aging in Christianity. In T. Cole, D. van Tassel and R. Kastenbaum (eds) *Handbook of the Humanities and Aging*. New York: Springer.

Pruitt, V. (1982) Yeats, the mask and the poetry of old age, *Journal of Geriatric Psychiatry*, 15(1), 99–112.

Radden, J. (1996) *Divided Minds and Successive Selves*. Cambridge, MA: MIT Press.

Ram-Prashad, C. (1995) A classical Indian philosophical perspective on ageing and the meaning of life, *Ageing and Society*, 15(1), 1–36.

Rawson, D. (1994) Models of interprofessional work. In A. Leathard (ed.) *Going Interprofessional: Working together for Health and Welfare*. London: Routledge.

Rechtschaffen, A. (1959) Psychotherapy with geriatric patients, *Journal of Gerontology*, 14, 73–84.

Rennemark, M. and Hagberg, B. (1997) Sense of coherence among the elderly in relation to their perceived life-history in an Eriksonian perspective, *Aging and Mental Health*, 1(3), 221–9.

Rennie, D. (1994) Storytelling in psychotherapy, *Psychotherapy*, 31, 234–43.

Rhodes, R. (1995) *The New Governance*. London: ESRC.

Rioch, M. (1970) The work of Wilfred Bion on groups, *Psychiatry*, 33, 21–33.

Riviere, J. (1929) Womanliness as a masquerade. In V. Burgin (ed.) *Formations of Fantasy*. London: Methuen.

Robbins, I. (1997) Understanding and treating of long term consequences of war trauma. In L. Hunt, M. Marshall and C. Rawlings (eds) *Past Trauma in Late Life*. London: Jessica Kingsley.

Roberts, V. (1994a) The organisation of work. In A. Obholzer and V. Roberts (eds) *The Unconscious at Work*. London: Routledge.

Roberts, V. (1994b) Till death do us part: caring and uncaring in work with the elderly. In A. Obholzer and V. Roberts (eds) *The Unconscious at Work*. London: Routledge.

Rubin, S. (1997) Self and object in the postmodern world, *Psychotherapy*, 34(1), 1–10.

Rustin, M. (1991) *The Good Society and the Inner World*. London: Verso.

Ruth, J. and Coleman, P. (1996) Personality and aging. In J. Birren and K. Schaic (eds) *Handbook of the Psychology of Aging*, 4th edn. New York: Academic Press.

Salaman, E. (1970) *A Collection of Moments*. London: Longman.

Samdersen, L. (1994) *Intimacy and Ageing*. Brisbane, QLD: ASG.

Samuels, A. (1984) Gender and psyche: developments in analytic psychology, *British Journal of Psychotherapy*, 1(1), 31–49.

Samuels, A. (1985) *Jung and the Post Jungians*. London: Routledge.

Samuels, A. (1993) *The Political Psyche*. London: Routledge.

Samuels, A., Shorter, B. and Plaut, F. (1986) *A Critical Dictionary of Jungian Analysis*. London: Routledge.

Sandywell, B. (1995) Forget Baudrillard? *Theory, Culture and Society*, 12, 125–52.

Sawchuk, K. (1995) From gloom to boom: age, identity and target marketing. In M. Featherstone and A. Wernick (eds) *Images of Ageing*. London: Routledge.

Sayers, J. (1994) Informal care and dementia: lessons for psychoanalysis and feminism, *Journal of Social Work Practice*, 8(2), 123–36.

Schroots, J. (1996) Theoretical developments in the psychology of aging, *The Gerontologist*, 36(6), 742–8.

Schutz, A. (1962) *Collected Works*. The Hague: Nijhoff.

Segal, H. (1958) Fear of death: notes on the analysis of an old man, *International Journal of Psychoanalysis*, 39(1), 178–81.

Sheehy, G. (1996) *New Passages: Mapping Your Life across Time*. New York: HarperCollins.

Sherman, E. and Webb, T. (1994) The self as a process in late life reminiscence; spiritual attributes, *Ageing and Society*, 14(2), 255–68.

Sinason, V. (1992) *Mental Handicap and the Human Condition*. London: Free Association Books.

Smart, B. (1993) *Postmodernity: Key Ideas*. London: Routledge.

Sparkes, T. (1994) A study of professional attitudes towards older people within an interprofessional context, *Journal of Interprofessional Care*, 8(2), 183–92.

Spence, D. (1986) Narrative smoothing and clinical wisdom. In T. Sarbin (ed.) *Narrative Psychology*. New York: Praeger.

Steinberg, D. (1992) Informed consent: consultation as a basis for collaboration between disciplines and between professionals and patients, *Journal of Interprofessional Care*, 6(1), 43–8.

Steiner, J. (1993) *Psychic Retreats*. London: Routledge.

Stevens, A. (1993) *To The Wellhouse*. London: CCETSW.

Stokes, J. (1994) Problems in multidisciplinary teams: the unconscious at work, *Journal of Social Work Practice*, 8(2), 161–8.

Sugarman, L. (1986) *Life-span Development*. London: Routledge.

Symington, J. and Symington, N. (1996) *The Clinical Thinking of Wilfred Bion*. London: Routledge.

Terry, P. (1997) *Counselling the Elderly and Their Carers*. London: Macmillan.

Terry, P. (1998) Who will care for older people? A case study of working with destructiveness and despair in long stay care, *Journal of Social Work Practice*. 12(2), 172–87.

Thompson, P. (1992) I don't feel old: subjective ageing and the search for meaning in later life, *Ageing and Society*, 12, 23–48.

Thompson, S. (1997) War experiences and post-traumatic stress disorder, *The Psychologist*, 10(8), 349–50.

Thursby, G. (1992) Islamic, Hindu and Buddhist conceptions of aging. In T. Cole, D. van Tassel and R. Kastenbaum (eds) *Handbook of Humanities and Aging*. New York: Springer.

Tornstam, L. (1994) Gero-transcendence: a theoretical and empirical investigation. In L. Thomas and S. Eisenhandler (eds) *Aging and the Religious Dimension*. Westport, CT: Auburn House.

Tornstam, L. (1996) Gerotranscendence: a theory about maturing into old age, *Journal of Aging and Identity*, 1(1), 37–50.

Town, N., Foster, R., Grant, S., Crosby, D., Emmerson, P., Williams, M., Edington, C. and Mountain, L. (1997) The County Durham users and carers forum, *Journal of Interprofessional Care*, 11(2), 139–48.

Townsend, P. (1963) *The Last Refuge*. London: Routledge.

Townsend, P. (1981) The structured dependency of the elderly: a creation of social policy in the twentieth century, *Ageing and Society*, 1(1), 5–28.

Townsend, P. (1986) Ageism and social policy. In C. Phillipson and A. Walker (eds) *Ageing and Social Policy*. London: Gower.

Tseelon, E. (1992) Is the presented self sincere? Goffman, impression management and the postmodern self, *Theory, Culture and Society*, 9, 115–28.

Tseelon, E. (1995) *The Masque of Femininity*. London: Sage.

Tudor, L. and Tudor, K. (1995) Acting up as acting out: containing anxiety in social services, *Changes*, 13, 241–52.

Turner, B. S. (1995) Aging and identity: some reflections on the somatisation of the self. In M. Featherstone and A. Wernick (eds) *Images of Ageing*. London: Routledge.

Twigg, J. and Aitkin, K. (1993) *Policy and Practice in Informal Care*. Buckingham: Open University Press.

Vaillant, G. (1993) *The Wisdom of the Ego*. Cambridge, MA: Harvard University Press.

van Deurzen-Smith, E. (1997) *Everyday Mysteries: Existential Dimensions of Psychotherapy*. London: Routledge.

van Geen, V. (1997) The measure and discuss intervention: a procedure for client empowerment and quality control in residential care homes, *The Gerontologist*, 37(6), 817–22.

Venn, C. (1997) Beyond enlightenment: after the subject of Foucault, who comes? *Theory, Culture and Society*, 14(3), 1–28.

Vialdi, A. (1996) Political identity and the transmission of trauma, *New Formations*, 30, 33–45.

von Kandratowitz, H.-J. (1998) *Developments in European Social Gerontology*. Helsinki: European Congress of Social Gerontology.

Walker, A. (1986) Pensions and the production of policy in old age. In C. Phillipson and A. Walker (eds) *Ageing and Social Policy*. Aldershot: Gower.

Ward, D. and Mullander, A. (1991) Empowerment and oppression: an indissoluble pairing for contemporary social work, *Critical Social Policy*, 32, 21–30.

Warnes, T., Boyle, S. and Hamblin, R. (1998) The most deprived inner city older population in Britain? *Generations Review*, 8(1), 8–10.

Weaver, R. (1973) *The Wise Old Woman*. Boston: Shambhala.

Webster, B. (1973) *Yeats: a Psychoanalytic Study*. London: Macmillan.

Williamson, J. (1978) *Decoding Advertisements*. London: Marion Boyars.

Wilson, G. (1991) Models of ageing and their relation to policy formation and service provision, *Policy and Politics*, 19(1), 37–47.

Woodhouse, D. and Pengelly, P. (1991) *Anxiety and the Dynamics of Collaboration*. Newcastle: Aberdeen University Press.

Woodward, K. (1991) *Aging and Its Discontents*. Bloomington, IN: Indiana University Press.

Woodward, K. (1995) Tribute to the older woman. In M. Featherstone and A. Wernick (eds) *Images of Ageing*. London: Routledge.

Woolfe, R. and Biggs, S. (1977) Counselling older adults: issues and awareness, *Counselling Psychology Quarterly*, 10(2), 189–94.

Woolger, R. (1987) *Other Lives, Other Selves*. New York: Crucible.

Yalom, I. (1980) *Existential Psychotherapy*. New York: Basic Books.

Zaretsky, E. (1997) Bisexuality, capitalism and the ambivalent legacy of psychoanalysis, *New Left Review*, 54, 69–89.

Index